Curriculum Development in Nursing Education

Carroll L. Iwasiw, RN, MScN, EdD
Professor and Former Director

Dolly Goldenberg, RN, MA (English), MScN, PhD
Professor and Chair, Graduate Programs

Mary-Anne Andrusyszyn, RN, MScN, EdD
Associate Professor

School of Nursing
Faculty of Health Sciences
University of Western Ontario
London, Ontario, Canada

JONES AND BARTLETT PUBLISHERS
Sudbury, Massachusetts
BOSTON   TORONTO   LONDON   SINGAPORE

World Headquarters
Jones and Bartlett Publishers
40 Tall Pine Drive
Sudbury, MA 01776
978-443-5000
info@jbpub.com
www.jbpub.com

Jones and Bartlett Publishers Canada
2406 Nikanna Road
Mississauga, ON L5C 2W6
CANADA

Jones and Bartlett Publishers International
Barb House, Barb Mews
London W6 7PA
UK

Library of Congress Cataloging-in-Publication Data

Iwasiw, Carroll.
    Curriculum development in nursing education / Carroll Iwasiw, Dolly Goldenberg, Mary-Anne Andrusyszyn.
        p. ; cm.
    Includes bibliographical references.
    ISBN 0-7637-2719-9 (pbk. : alk. paper)
  1. Nursing—Study and teaching. 2. Curriculum planning.
    [DNLM: 1. Education, Nursing. 2. Curriculum. WY 18 I96c 2005] I. Goldenberg, Dolly. II. Andrusyszyn, Mary-Anne. III. Title.
    RT71.I95 2005
    610.73′071′1—dc22

                                    2004021351

Production Credits
Acquisitions Editor: Kevin Sullivan
Production Manager: Amy Rose
Associate Editor: Amy Sibley
Production Assistant: Kate Hennessy
Associate Marketing Manager: Emily Ekle
Manufacturing and Inventory Coordinator: Amy Bacus
Composition: Auburn Associates, Inc.
Cover Design: Timothy Dziewit
Printing and Binding: Malloy Inc.
Cover Printing: Malloy Inc.

Printed in the United States of America
08 07 06 05   10 9 8 7 6 5 4 3 2

Preface

This book has been a venture of dedication and purpose. As nursing education faculty and teachers of curriculum development for a number of years, we endeavored to write an entire textbook specifically on curriculum development.

This book is about the processes of curriculum development. We do not advocate any particular curriculum philosophy, model, design, teaching approach, or evaluation strategy. Rather, we propose ideas for creating a curriculum. This book offers a current, accessible, and comprehensive text on curriculum development, and incorporates a balance of theoretical perspectives and practical applications. There is some reference to historical beginnings, providing context for traditional, new, and emerging ideas. The book is written for all those who engage in designing or developing nursing curricula in baccalaureate, associate degree, and diploma nursing education, such as recently appointed or experienced nurse faculty as well as part-time and adjunct faculty, graduate students, teaching assistants, and those who aspire to become nurse educators. Other health professionals may also benefit.

Few textbooks of this nature have been printed in the past two decades, apart from the 3rd edition of E. O. Bevis's *Curriculum Building in Nursing: A Process* (1982/86/89). Helpful information on curriculum development, nonetheless, has been available from nursing education literature, from the National League for Nursing, and from chapters in nursing education textbooks written by nurse scholars.

The practice of nursing education is changing, due to ongoing developments in the fields of general education, nursing education, and health care. Socio-cultural-political forces, a shifting market and global-driven economy, nurse and nurse-faculty shortages, changing values, and life's uncertainties also impinge upon how we prepare graduates for their nursing practice and educative roles. Information and health care technologies, creative delivery methods, culturally diverse student groups, nursing education as a science, and evidence-based teaching are additional issues nursing faculty must face. These factors must be considered in curriculum development.

We have used the term *nursing curriculum* to mean the totality of the curriculum: philosophical approaches, goals, design, courses, teaching and evaluation strategies, and outcomes; interactions and learning climate; human and physical resources; and curriculum policies. Throughout the book, the term *student clinical experience* is used to refer to practice experiences in all health care and community contexts: acute-care hospitals, long-term care facilities, walk-in clinics, private practitioners' offices, public health agencies, day-care facilities, people's homes, store-front clinics, and so forth. The term *clinical* is inclusive of the full range of practice experiences and sites possible in a nursing curriculum.

The process of curriculum development is iterative, with many phases taking place concurrently. However, for purposes of structure, the book has been organized into 11 chapters. Effort has been made throughout the book to refer readers to previous and subsequent chapters to facilitate conceptual links. Considerable thought has been given in the first six chapters to early curriculum development activities, phases in the curriculum process worthy of attention. Fictionalized case studies have been included in each chapter to highlight the main ideas, and to assist readers in deliberations pertaining to related curriculum development activities. Questions are included in each chapter to stimulate thinking about curriculum development in your setting.

Chapter 1 introduces curriculum development in nursing. Chapter 2 offers some preliminary considerations for undertaking the curriculum development process, while Chapter 3 outlines some practical considerations for getting organized. The importance of faculty development is introduced early in the book, and Chapter 4 concentrates on faculty development related to curriculum development. This becomes an important component of succeeding chapters. Chapter 5 addresses gathering data about contextual factors that influence curriculum development, and this is followed by an entirely new perspective in Chapter 6, determining curriculum directions from the contextual data. The philosophical approaches and goals that form the basis of the curriculum comprise Chapter 7. Conceptual frameworks have not been considered separately, as we view these to be part of the philosophical approaches. Curriculum design is presented in Chapter 8, and course design in Chapter 9. Planning for curriculum evaluation, albeit an activity which is ongoing during curriculum development, comprises Chapter 10. Finally, in Chapter 11, planning for curriculum implementation offers important considerations sometimes overlooked when developing nursing curricula.

The book is unique in its concentrated presentation of the ways and means of curriculum development in nursing education. If you are already involved in this activity, this book may stimulate reflection on your current curriculum development approaches as well as provide some additional perspectives. If you are new to curriculum development, the book will make you a more informed participant in this process.

Acknowledgments

We would like to thank all our professors and those nursing leaders who have been inspirational to us in writing this textbook: Professors Em Olivia Bevis, Mildred Gottdank, Shirley-Jo Paine, Dorothy Reilly, and Vivian Wood. They have stimulated our interest in, respect for, and dedication to nursing education. We also thank the graduate students in our nursing education courses whose discussion and questions extended our thinking about curriculum development. We dedicate this book to you.

We are grateful to our families, colleagues, and friends, for their encouragement throughout this endeavor. In particular, Zenon Andrusyszyn for his graphics and sustaining support, Dr. Sol Goldenberg for his wit and humor, and Mary Iwasiw for her enduring confidence. We also thank those at Jones and Bartlett who helped bring this book to publication.

Table of Contents

3
Organizing for Curriculum Development:
The Practical Considerations

4
Faculty Development and Change for
Curriculum Development

8
Curriculum Design   165

10
Planning Curriculum Evaluation

11
Planning for Successful Curriculum Implementation 243

CHAPTER 1

Introduction to Curriculum Development in Nursing Education

Curriculum development is an ongoing activity in nursing education, even in established curricula. The extent of the development ranges from regular refinement of class activities and assignments to the creation of a completely new curriculum. In this book, curriculum development activities are presented individually for ease of description and comprehension. The authors underscore their view that the curriculum development process does not necessarily occur in stages or phases, because some work occurs simultaneously and each new decision has the potential to affect previous ones. This chapter contains a summary of the major aspects of the curriculum development process, serving as an advance organizer for the book. Additionally, attention is given to some of the interpersonal issues that can influence the curriculum development team, and hence, the completed work. The ideas about curriculum development presented in this chapter are discussed more expansively in succeeding chapters.

Curriculum

Definitions of *curriculum* have been in existence since about 1820, first used in Scotland and then professionally in America a century later (Wiles & Bondi, 1998). There have been so many definitions, often in response to social forces, that the scope and interpretation of curriculum have not only greatly expanded, but possibly created some uncertainty and divergence of opinion as to meaning or intent. This "very breadth may make the definition nonfunctional," but limiting [it] "might be too confining to be adequate for modern [usage]" (Taba, 1962, p. 9).

From the more traditional definition of a *course of study*, to *a program of planned, unplanned, technical and practical ranges of experiences*, to *interactions between and among teachers and students for learning to take place*, curriculum has also been conceived as legitimate (sanctioned), illegitimate (not sanctioned), hidden (socialized), and null (thought, but not there) (Bevis, 2000; Eisner, 1985). It may also have taken on meaning according to educators' individual and collective values and beliefs about education, teaching, and learning.

The position taken by R. C. Doll is that curriculum can be improvable in content and process, formally and informally, to the extent that learners gain knowledge, understanding, attitudes, appreciation, and values. More conceptually, W. E. Doll Jr. described curriculum in relation to a shifting paradigm, moving from a formal definition to a focus on multiple interactions with people and surroundings (Dillard, Siktberg, & Laidig, 2005).

Despite differing conceptions, a curriculum usually contains philosophical statements and goals, indicates some selection, organization and sequencing of subject matter, and integrates evaluation. These elements, among others, are addressed in this book. The authors view the term *nursing curriculum* to mean the totality of the curriculum goals, design, courses, teaching and evaluation strategies, and outcomes; interactions and learning climate; human and physical resources; and curriculum policies.

Curriculum Development in Nursing Education

Curriculum development is a process that can be described as more akin to art than science. It is characterized by interaction, cooperation, change, and possibly conflict; comprised of overlapping, interactive, and iterative decisions; shaped by contextual realities and political timeliness; and influenced by personal interests, philosophies, judgments, and values. The complex processes that lead to the creation of a curriculum provide an opportunity for faculty members to develop and implement new perspectives on the education of nursing students and to influence the culture of the school of nursing. As well, curriculum development provides an avenue to strengthen the school's impact on the community and gain support from members of the educational institution, community, and nursing profession.

The Curriculum Development Process

Curriculum development has no beginning nor end, and there is no perfect product for the final curriculum document. Scales (1985) wrote that "in actual practice, development and implementation of the curriculum is an integrated phenomenon . . . developed in a very integrated and interrelating manner; one component . . . not necessarily spring[ing] full grown and naturally from another, nor will any single component usually stand without some revision after subsequent parts are developed" (p. 3). Her view of curriculum development as an iterative process is repeated throughout this textbook.

Although written and schematic representations of curriculum development are generally linear and sequential, this is not how curricula are developed in reality, as noted above. Curriculum development is a highly iterative process, with each decision influencing concurrent choices and possibly causing a rethinking of previous ideas. A unified curriculum results from ongoing communication among groups working on different aspects of curriculum development, review and critique of completed work, and confirmation of decisions. Faculty development activities during development, implementation, and evaluation of the curriculum prepare faculty to influence the curriculum through knowledgeable participation. The model of the curriculum development process in nursing education, which is described in this book, is illustrated in Figure 1.1 and summarized below.

Determine Need for Change The creation of a new curriculum begins with acknowledging that the existing curriculum is no longer working as effectively as desired. This recognition can arise from altered circumstances within the school (e.g., changing faculty or student profile), or outside the school (e.g., changed standards of nursing practice or accreditation standards). Although the need for change may be readily apparent to some faculty members, others may resist the idea of curriculum change.

Gain Support Curriculum change cannot occur without the support of faculty and administrators. Gaining support for the curriculum development enterprise includes describing the logical reasons for altering the curriculum and appealing to the values held collectively by members of the school and educational institution. Faculty members' support and commitment are essential for all curriculum endeavors. Additionally, administrative support, in the form of altered work assignments, secretarial assistance, and possibly promotion and tenure considerations, provides evidence of institutional encouragement for the initiative. Those persons desirous of curriculum change need to ensure that the means to complete the work will be available. Without assurance of such resources, faculty members are hesitant to undertake curriculum development. Additionally, support from nursing leaders, clinicians, and other stakeholders is essential.

Organize for Curriculum Change Attention to the logistical matters that will lead to a successful outcome is essential. Organizing for curriculum change requires consideration of and decisions about leadership, the decision-making processes, committee structures and purposes, and approaches to getting the work done. Determining a critical path for curriculum development is a valuable strategy to ensure that deadlines for milestones in the process are known and met.

Plan and Implement Faculty Development Faculty development is essential throughout the curriculum development process. Although curriculum development is inherently a faculty development activity, some members of the curriculum development team may need

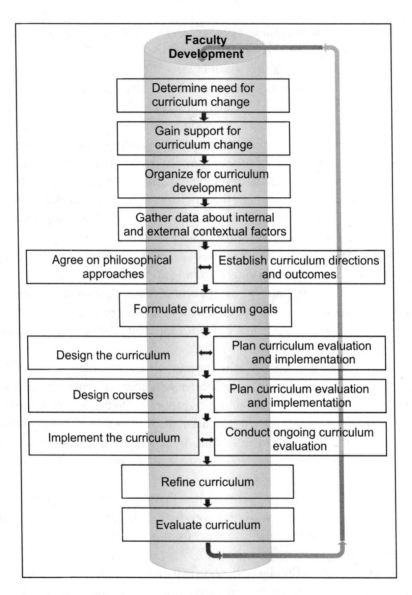

Figure 1.1 Curriculum Development Model

more definitive assistance to acquire the knowledge and skills necessary to engage in curriculum work. Accordingly, faculty development should occur in concert with curriculum development, preparing members for each aspect of the process. To support new philosophical, teaching, and delivery approaches, ongoing faculty development is necessary during curriculum implementation.

Gather Data About Internal and External Contextual Factors Systematic data-gathering is critical to ensure that the curriculum is relevant for the environment in which graduates will practice nursing. Contextual factors are those forces, situations, and circumstances that exist both within and outside the educational institution and have the potential to influence the school and its programs. Internal contextual factors exist within the school and the educational institution; external contextual factors originate outside the institution.

Typically, information is obtained about internal factors of history; philosophy, mission, and goals; culture; financial resources; programs and policies; and infrastructure. External contextual factors are: demographics; culture; health care; professional standards and trends; technology; environment; and socio-politico-economics. These factors are inter-related, complex, and at times seamless and overlapping. Therefore, it is necessary to determine precisely which data are required about each of the factors.

Agree on Philosophical Approaches Information about philosophical approaches used in nursing education, along with faculty values and beliefs, leads to the development of statements of philosophical approaches relevant for the school and curriculum. Reaching resolution about the philosophical approaches is a critical milestone in curriculum development, since all aspects of the finalized curriculum should be congruent with espoused values and beliefs.

Determine Curriculum Directions and Outcomes Decisions about curriculum directions and outcomes are also highly important in curriculum development. These arise from an analysis and synthesis of the contextual data. This synthesis involves reviewing the contextual data; proposing important concepts, competencies, potential designs, and possible learning activities; and identifying limitations for the curriculum as well as administrative issues that could affect the curriculum. From this integrative thinking and the philosophical approaches, ideas are developed about important outcomes for program graduates and the design of the curriculum.

Formulate Curriculum Goals Curriculum goals are written to incorporate the outcomes, philosophical approaches, and predominant concepts in the curriculum. The goals reflect broad abilities of graduates, each representing an integration of cognitive, psychomotor, and/or affective actions. The goals are a public statement of what program graduates will be like.

Design the Curriculum The term *curriculum design* refers to the configuration of the course of studies. In designing the curriculum, faculty determine level goals; nursing, support, and elective courses; their sequencing; the relationships between and among courses; delivery methods; and associated policies. Brief course descriptions and general course goals are prepared for nursing courses.

Design Courses Course design requires attention to the following components: purpose and description, goals, teaching strategies, content, classes, student learning activities, and evaluation of student learning. Each course must be congruent with the curriculum intent and clearly relate to curriculum goals.

Plan Evaluation Curriculum evaluation is an organized and thoughtful appraisal of those elements central to the course of studies undertaken by students and of the abilities of graduates. The aspects to be evaluated include the curriculum goals, design, and outcomes; courses; teaching and evaluation strategies; human and physical resources; learning climate; and curriculum policies. Planning curriculum evaluation should occur simultaneously with curriculum and course design.

Plan Implementation Successful implementation of the curriculum is dependent on forethought as the curriculum is being designed. Informing stakeholders, marketing, attending to contractual agreements and logistics, and planning ongoing faculty development are essential aspects of preparing for implementation.

Interpersonal Aspects of Curriculum Development

Curriculum development is not a sterile process of objective, detached decision-making. Rather, it is marked by the dynamics of all interpersonal activities. As such, learning, conflict, cooperation, resistance, eagerness, formation of group alliances, commitment to shared goals, sadness, and satisfaction can occur. The human dimension is a constant factor in curriculum development, and must be attended to even when the tasks of curriculum development are pressing. It is important, therefore, to ensure that all members of the curriculum development team feel valued and appreciated for ideas they offer and work they complete.

Curriculum deliberations occur in collaboration with colleagues whose perspectives, conclusions, and values may be divergent. Values affect the choices people make and the perceptions they place on attitudes, ideals, attributes, and objects (Hamilton, 1992). Accordingly, values are a powerful influence on curriculum development and it is incumbent upon curriculum developers to reflect on their values. Therefore, values clarification is integral to curriculum development, and can be essential in times of emotional debate or apparently irresolvable conflict.

Resistance to curriculum change can occur because of differing values about nursing education, feelings of uncertainty about fitting into a new curriculum, disinterest, or a general disinclination to expend the effort necessary to create and implement a new curriculum. Such resistance can sabotage the efforts of committed curricularists and may require intervention by colleagues and the dean or director. Implementation of strategies to overcome resistance can be important throughout curriculum development and implementation.

Creating and implementing a new curriculum represent a significant change for faculty in which they progress from known and comfortable ways of being, to uncertainty, to new understandings and practices. Curriculum change requires collegial support and reinforcement. Collectively, faculty can implement strategies to recognize their progress, offer encouragement to each other, and celebrate their successes. In these ways, both faculty cohesion and the curriculum are strengthened.

A full review of interpersonal dynamics is beyond the scope of this book. However, diligent attention should be given to this aspect of curriculum development. The success of the curriculum is dependent on the dedication of all stakeholders and this is most likely to develop when individuals communicate openly and supportively with one another.

Chapter Summary

Curriculum development is an endeavor that faculty and other stakeholders undertake with the goal of creating a program whose graduates will practice nursing competently in a constantly changing health care environment. It begins with the recognition that the existing curriculum does not meet established purposes and goals, and formally concludes when the new curriculum is implemented. However, curriculum development is really an ongoing process, since evaluation and revision are constant features of nursing programs. Successful curriculum development is contingent on dedicated faculty who feel valued for their efforts and who are supported during personal transition and change.

References

Bevis, E.O. (2000). Nursing curriculum as professional education. In E.O. Bevis & J. Watson (Eds.), *Toward a caring curriculum. A new pedagogy for nursing.* (pp. 67–106). Boston: Jones and Bartlett Publishers.

Dillard, N., Sikterg, L., & Laidig, J. (2005). Curriculum development: An overview. In D.M. Billings & J.A. Halstead (Eds.), *Teaching in nursing. A guide for faculty.* (pp 87-107). Philadelphia: Elsevier Saunders.

Eisner, E. (1985). *The educational imagination* (2nd ed.). New York: MacMillan.

Hamilton, P.M. (1992). *Realities of contemporary nursing.* Menlo Park, CA: Addison-Wesley Nursing.

Scales, F.S. (1985). *Nursing curriculum. Development, structure, function.* Norwalk, CT: Appleton-Century Crofts.

Taba, H. (1962). *Curriculum development. Theory and practice.* New York: Harcourt Brace Yovanovich, Inc.

Wiles, J., & Bondi, J. (1998). *Curriculum development. A guide to practice* (5th ed.). Upper Saddle River, N.J.: Merrill.

CHAPTER 2

Preliminary Considerations for Curriculum Development

Chapter Overview

This chapter provides insight into considerations that must precede a decision to undertake curriculum development, either from the perspective of designing a new curriculum or of revising an existing one. Although a revision or a completely new curriculum may seem the obvious choice for rectifying some aspect of a program, it is worthwhile to carefully consider faculty willingness to undertake this endeavor. Reflection about the reasons for curriculum change, who will be involved, the timeframe, and how to gain support for the idea are addressed. A chapter summary follows. Synthesis activities include two cases: the first is followed by a critique, and the second provides an opportunity to analyze readiness for curriculum revision or development. Questions to guide thinking about preliminary considerations for curriculum development conclude the chapter. These questions are designed to help the reader decide if circumstances are right to begin the formal process of curriculum development in individual settings.

Chapter Goals

- Consider factors and influences that precipitate curriculum development or revision
- Identify participants in the curriculum development process
- Assess acceptance of and readiness for curriculum development or revision
- Justify the decision to proceed with or suspend the curriculum development process

Considerations for Curriculum Development

Why Consider Curriculum Change?

The purpose of nursing programs is to graduate nurses who will contribute to the health and quality of life of individuals and the community they serve. Situations that impede the ability of the school of nursing to achieve this purpose, and consequently threaten its stability, success, or reputation, precipitate thoughts of curriculum change. Among such circumstances could be alterations in:

- success rates on licensure or registration examinations
- accreditation or approval standards
- institutional, professional, and/or governmental regulations
- new graduates' ability to meet employers' expectations
- resources available in the school of nursing
- faculty numbers or expertise
- educational technologies
- competition from other schools
- organization of nursing education, state- or province-wide
- nursing workforce
- provision of health care
- nursing and educational paradigms

Trends, demographics, local and national circumstances, economics, technologies, professional priorities, changing values and beliefs about teaching and learning, nursing, and nursing education, are all interrelated conditions to which nursing curricula must respond (Bevis, 2000a; Bowen, Lyons, & Young, 2000; Conley, 1973). As well, the desire for curriculum change can arise from a generalized discontent with the status quo and a desire to replace old ideas with new ones. Members of the school of nursing may identify learning gaps in the existing curriculum when personal and professional ideologies of nursing and health care shift, when advances are made in educational technology, or when new ideas are introduced by incoming faculty.

Additionally, the impetus for curriculum change may be a groundswell for profound changes in nursing curricula, such as has been proclaimed for many years (Bevis, 2000a,b; Bevis & Clayton, 1988; Diekelmann, 1997; Freeman, Voignier, & Scott, 2002; Heller, Oros, & Durney-Crowley, 2000; Howell Adams et al., 2001; Lindeman, 2000; Moccia, 1990; Watson, 2000a,b). Curriculum reconceptualization, revision, and/or development is a continuing process in most nursing programs. " . . . Nurse educators, sensitive to the increasingly evident inadequacies of current educational thinking are evaluating their belief systems, redefining their curriculum approaches and altering their teaching practices. . . ." (Attridge, 1996, p. 406). In fact, the most significant change in nursing education in the last 10 years, according to Pesut (as cited in Pesut, 1995) is the "transformation of the problem-focused nursing process model into a more sophisticated outcome-oriented, clinical decision and reasoning model" (p. 9).

Outdated methods and assumptions of educating nursing students are being re-examined and replaced in light of changing perspectives and the abilities required for nurses of today and tomorrow. Contemporary nursing curricula must be designed with critical and creative requisites for nursing practice.

> . . . nursing philosophy and theory and nursing education have come to a crossroads. Critical and ethical thinking, creativity . . . liberating curriculum from restrictive methodologies, grounding education in the realities of practice . . . caring [which is] . . . reoriented toward a new vision of the whole person [must] pervade the curriculum . . . (Graubard, 2000, p.xiii).

Why is curriculum change necessary? Why revise or implement new curricula? The simple and most direct answer is that contemporary environments require it. In other words, because we must. We owe it to students, graduates, the community, and society at large. Dramatic shifts in health and in the health care system, in technologies, in population profiles, expectations, and demands have led to the realization that the education of nurses, and therefore our curricula, must be subjected to re-evaluation, revision, and maybe even dramatic change. Oermann's (1995) conviction for change is evident when she writes, "Nursing education is being forced to deal realistically with broad human issues within the context of care delivery and a redefinition of health . . . health care cannot be effectively rendered outside the cultural and psychological realities of individuals and their communities . . ." (p. 8). The magnitude, pace, and intensity of these dynamic changes challenge nurse educators to develop more relevant and evidence-based curricula to prepare nurses for new roles and responsibilities consistent with the evolving health care system. A curriculum is a living, dynamic entity, so change is inevitable.

How and Where Will Support Be Gained?

Faculty desiring curriculum change should seek support from every source imaginable: learners, faculty, clinical colleagues, health care clients, and administrators. The support of representatives from each group strengthens the case for proceeding with curriculum development work. However, at this early stage, initial support is needed from faculty colleagues and the dean or director of the school of nursing so that the intensive work can be formally started. It also is helpful to identify possible funding sources for curriculum development, such as internal university funds or foundations known to support innovation in nursing education.

It is essential to clearly articulate why curriculum development is necessary. For example, it is important to present factual data about how deficiencies in the current curriculum are evident (e.g., failure rate on licensing exams). Similarly, the changing trends that led to the conclusion that the curriculum is outdated should be addressed.

Gaining support for curriculum development involves an appeal to logic and values. Neither one alone is sufficient. The precise approach will, of course, be dependent on the organization and the people involved. The educational institution might pride itself on being innovative, responsive to diversity, and a leader in education. If so, linking the concept of curriculum change with these prized values will help "sell" the idea. In Table 2.1, suggestions are offered which will be helpful in convincing others that curriculum development is needed.

It is important to consider the best way to seek support. Should colleagues be approached individually or collectively? Clearly, there are advantages and drawbacks to both (See Table 2.2 for an analysis of approaching colleagues individually or collectively). A combination may be appropriate, first talking with colleagues individually to gain the acceptance of informal leaders, and then presenting ideas to a larger group. The decision will be influenced by knowledge of the interpersonal dynamics among colleagues and by the credibility of those seeking support for curriculum change.

The support of the dean or director is necessary before curriculum work can proceed, no matter how much endorsement exists among faculty. Matters to address with the school leader are included in Table 2.3. It is unlikely that precise information about each point will be available. However, recognition of both the academic and administrative aspects of curriculum development will increase credibility with the head of the nursing program.

How Can Initial Objections Be Addressed?

Overcoming Objections Initial resistance is an expected reaction to the possibility of change. Overcoming initial objections to the idea of curriculum development is an important

TABLE 2.1   SUGGESTIONS TO CONVINCE OTHERS OF NEED FOR CURRICULUM CHANGE

Appeal to Logic	Appeal to Values
Need for curriculum change or development due to: • deficiency in current curriculum • trends requiring new approaches • evidence from literature to support change Requirement to provide a curriculum responsive to health care and societal needs Need for curriculum to be congruent with mission, values of organization Possibility of obtaining funding for curriculum development	Congruence with: • organizational mission and values • personal and professional values Desire for: • professional and personal growth of learners • competent graduates • enhancement of School prestige • status as innovators, leaders Opportunity for: • personal prestige • innovation and transformation • organizational preeminence • enhanced reputation Consequences of avoiding curriculum development: • decreased appeal and marketability of School to students, faculty, and employers of graduates • lost opportunities for funding • implications for accreditation • diminished prestige

part of winning support. (Responding to ongoing resistance to curriculum change is addressed in Chapter 4.) To ignore initial opposition may result in failure to proceed. Therefore, it is essential to anticipate, recognize, and respond to objections promptly.

First, challenges about the accuracy of information that illustrates the need for curriculum change, or the conclusions drawn, can be anticipated. This may reflect an honest, intellectual disagreement; a deeply held belief in the value of the current curriculum; a general response to change; or opposition to the one advocating curriculum change.

TABLE 2.2   ADVANTAGES AND DISADVANTAGES OF APPROACHING COLLEAGUES
INDIVIDUALLY OR COLLECTIVELY

Approach	Advantages	Disadvantages
Individual	Freer expression and exploration of ideas	One viewpoint; no collective ideas
	Less threatening	Lack of support for persons proposing change
	Quick response or possible decision	Time required to collect and compile ideas from individuals
	Greater willingness to share experiences	Discomfort resulting from disagreement
	In-depth, thoughtful response possible	Pressure to conform
	Personal consultation valued	
Collective	Group response more broad	Delayed response or decision (many ideas before consensus)
	Sharing of many ideas	
	Opportunity to use democratic or consensual process, which strengthens a decision to proceed	Time required to share all experiences relative to decision
		Potential group veto of curriculum change
	Increased awareness of others' strengths and weaknesses	Undue influence by strong group members
	Opportunity to learn from each others' feedback	Group think
	Improved faculty bonding by uniting to reach common goal	
	Shared thinking for responses, resulting in a stronger position	
	Less time-consuming	
	Opportunity for group to make more informed assessments of need for change	

TABLE 2.3   MATTERS TO DISCUSS WITH SCHOOL LEADER

1. Need for curriculum change

2. Extent of colleague support

3. Estimated time for development and implementation of new or revised curriculum

4. Effect on other work:
   - teaching (classroom, clinical)
   - student advisement
   - research, publications, presentations
   - committee and community involvement

5. People to be involved

6. Resources needed:
   - faculty release time
   - support personnel
   - materials
   - technological equipment
   - physical space
   - funding

When reasons for curriculum change are questioned, it is tempting to invite challengers to explain their position. This is a strategy to be used with caution. Involvement in a distracting and ongoing dispute about who is right is not productive. It could lead to criticism by those who feel that their current teaching is the real work of the school of nursing. It is more constructive to respond that the reasons are compelling but, naturally, all will draw their own conclusions.

It may be that people are feeling overstretched so that even the idea of curriculum development, and thus more work, is overwhelming. The time required for this endeavor can seem daunting and may be a real barrier. It is important to acknowledge that curriculum development is a large undertaking. The reality of workloads and time available should be explored thoroughly: competing demands may make curriculum development impossible at this time. Perhaps some responsibilities can be delayed or given up, at least for a short period, to allow the process to unfold.

To win the support of particular individuals, it is wise to identify the criticisms they have voiced about the current curriculum, as well as aspects they value. Through individual or small group meetings, they can be reminded that curriculum development is an opportunity to eliminate the weaker aspects of the current curriculum. As well, it is essential to emphasize that their active involvement in the curriculum development process could lead to incorporating parts of the curriculum they cherish. Affirming that strengths of the present curriculum may be retained, if this is deemed appropriate, might induce cooperation.

Financial constraints will be a concern for the school leader. Curriculum development takes time, and faculty and staff time is costly. It is necessary, therefore, to enumerate the costs and potential risks of avoiding curriculum development. These can include unfavorable external reviews by approval or accrediting bodies, decreased ability to attract students and faculty, difficulty retaining faculty, and unrealized funding opportunities. Ideas for managing curriculum development will go a long way in gaining support.

Another reason for objecting to the idea of curriculum development might be that those proposing curriculum change do not have the respect of colleagues. The same idea, introduced by others, could be well received. Identifying if personalities are the reason why the idea of curriculum development is not supported, is a painful process. Those advocating curriculum change might consider whether or not their ideas are usually sought and supported by colleagues and if others generally choose to work with them. If personality seems to be a reason for objecting to the idea of curriculum development, it may be wise to leave the initiation of curriculum development to others. If this is not possible, some interpersonal work must be done before support will be gained for curriculum change. Table 2.4 summarizes objections that may be raised to the idea of curriculum revision or development, and offers possible responses.

Not all objections will be overcome, nor will all resistance melt away. Nonetheless, once a majority of faculty agrees with the need for curriculum change and the dean or director is supportive, the curriculum development process is ready to proceed. Faculty support for curriculum development is the foundation upon which the quality of the curriculum will rest.

Who Should Be Involved?

Curriculum development does not take place in a vacuum within an educational institution. Rather, many others in addition to faculty should be involved in the process. The education of nurses (and therefore, the development of curriculum) should not be the exclusive right or responsibility of academics (Carmon, Hauber, & Chase, 1992). In fact, Bevis (2000b) goes so far as to say that anyone "out there in the real world . . . . [and in] nursing or health care" (p. 114), should be included in curriculum development. In her seminal work, *Curriculum and Instruction in Nursing*, Conley (1973) wrote that individuals or groups who exert some influence, directly or indirectly, should have some determination for the nature and activi-

TABLE 2.4   RESPONSES TO INITIAL OBJECTIONS TO THE IDEA OF CURRICULUM CHANGE

Nature of Objections	Responses
Challenge to reasons for curriculum change	Respond that reasons are compelling
Satisfaction with current curriculum	Emphasize the: • importance of offering a curriculum that will maximize student learning and graduates' success • opportunity to be on the cutting edge of change and transformation in nursing education • personal and professional growth potential inherent in curriculum development
Fear that treasured part of the curriculum will be lost	Affirm that as curriculum work proceeds, aspects of the current curriculum may be retained Comment that active involvement is the only means to ensure a satisfactory curriculum
Time required for curriculum development	Present possible funding opportunities for curriculum development and faculty release time Note that individuals' involvement will influence process, and thus, time required
Fear that curriculum development will negatively affect research and writing time	Underscore the opportunities for research and scholarly writing that arise from curriculum development, implementation, and evaluation State that curriculum development is a role responsibility
Lack of support for faculty proposing change	Let credible faculty initiate idea of curriculum change

ties of the curriculum. The parent institution, the larger community, and society at large have a role to play in the design and implementation of the nursing curriculum. More specifically, concerted efforts of administrators, consumers, practitioners, students, and faculty are required.

Nonetheless, shaping curriculum is very much the province of the faculty. Faculty have the most direct influence on curriculum development by virtue of their knowledge, experience, and decision-making power (Conley, 1973). Indeed, curriculum development is the pivotal and ongoing point of the faculty's activities in most nursing programs (Rush, Ouellet, & Wasson, 1991). However, curriculum development is not only the responsibility of those teaching in the curriculum undergoing change; faculty in all programs ought to participate, as should the school leader.

Student participation in curriculum development is also very important (Thornton & Chapman, 2000). Students bring previous experiences and perspectives, needs and aspirations, which when combined, influence the curriculum. Their role in curriculum development should be as credible as that of other participants (Attridge, 1996).

The importance of collaborative interfacing with colleagues from practice settings should not be overlooked. Service agencies are affected by the curriculum and potential faculty role changes. Clinical experts can provide useful, practical input, and validate suggested practice changes. Curriculum dialogue among faculty, students, administrators, and clinicians has been described as mutually enriching, not only to themselves, but to the curriculum and profession (Carmon et al., 1992).

Who else should be involved in the curriculum development process? When writing about the curriculum revolution, Rentschler and Spegman (1996) include anyone from the larger community, and suggest that these individuals might also serve on curriculum advisory boards. Such stakeholders could include faculty from other disciplines, program graduates, professors emeriti, health care leaders, educators from the school system, community leaders, and clients, as well as members of professional bodies. Their knowledge, experience, and vested interests would assure that standards are maintained, and expectations of preparing nurses "for the changing health care field, rapid proliferation of health knowledge and technology, and diverse client needs" (p. 390) are upheld. Table 2.5 represents those who should be involved in curriculum development.

What Will the Timeframe Be?

An important consideration when undertaking curriculum revision or development of an entirely new curriculum is the timeframe for conclusion of the work. How urgent is the curriculum change and when does it need to be completed? There are several factors to examine when thinking about the start and completion dates for the potential curriculum development project. Each must be assessed within the context of all the other questions posed in this chapter.

First is the urgency of the curriculum change. This is influenced by the factors that prompted consideration of a change in the first place. If, for example, graduates for several years have had a high failure rate on licensing examinations, then improving the curriculum is urgent and faculty must complete curriculum changes quickly. Similarly, a change in clinical services in local health care agencies may necessitate an immediate refocusing of clini-

TABLE 2.5   PERSONS INVOLVED IN CURRICULUM DEVELOPMENT

Graduate and undergraduate nursing faculty

Nursing students

Nursing dean or director

Program graduates

Professors emeriti

Educational institution administrators

Health care leaders

Clinicians

Professional nursing association members

Community leaders

Clients

Faculty in related and non-related disciplines

Educators from the school system

cal courses. Conversely, the immediacy of altering an undergraduate curriculum to reflect a slowly changing trend in local demographics is not as great.

Another factor to review when contemplating a timeframe is the culture of the organization. Is this an organization that innovates, or one that is satisfied with the status quo? Does it operate at a measured pace, with each step clearly delineated, or is implementation expected to rapidly follow decisions (Tappan, 2001)? Will it be necessary to gain approval from administrators for each step of the curriculum development process, or will they want only to be informed of progress? The speed at which work normally proceeds within the organization will affect the interval allotted for curriculum change.

The normal work cycle of the organization influences the schedule for beginning and completing the curriculum development process. Is there a semester when faculty are normally less busy with implementing programs and able to devote concentrated time to curriculum development? If so, consider how much work could be achieved in those time periods. If not, analyze the amount of curriculum development time that can be integrated into the ongoing work of the school.

Finally, when thinking about a timeframe for curriculum development, a mindful review should be conducted of the people who will be involved to identify those likely to be supporters and resisters. How much time can the supporters be expected to give to curriculum development? How much time will be taken up with overcoming resistance and winning support? This too will impact the expected completion of the curriculum. Before trying to gain support for curriculum development, it is important to have a schedule in mind. Participants must have some idea of the amount of time and work that is being asked of them before they can commit to a curriculum project.

Chapter Summary

Complex, interrelated factors need to be considered before decisions are made to embark on curriculum development. Paying attention to who might be involved and the timeframe for curriculum development will influence the ability to gain support for curriculum change and to move the process forward. The impetus and decision to proceed must be thoughtfully reviewed, since the process of curriculum development is intensive, extensive, and requires ongoing involvement and support of stakeholders. Commitment to the process must be a value shared by all participants.

Synthesis Activities

Two case studies are presented to illustrate the ideas of this chapter. The first is critiqued. Consider whether pertinent aspects of the case have been assessed and whether there are other points to be discussed. The second case is followed by questions to guide analysis. Finally, questions are offered for consideration of curriculum change in your situation.

Charlevoix University Undergraduate Nursing Program

Charlevoix University School of Nursing has introduced a new integrated baccalaureate-nursing program. The final year includes a classroom course and an associated clinical course about nursing of clients with complex needs. Broad goals and general descriptions for the courses were developed by the curriculum designers. Tom McLean, a clinical nurse specialist in the intensive care unit of a quaternary-care teaching hospital, was hired to design and teach the classroom course and manage the associated clinical course.

These courses are intended to help students integrate concepts from other nursing and support courses in situations of high acuity related to physiological, psychological, and/or social needs. Tom developed the classroom and clinical courses mainly by himself, consulting with the Undergraduate Program Chair about matters related to course structure: hours of instruction, regulations about examinations, frequency of clinical evaluation, and so forth. In his first year of teaching, Tom's content focus in the course was the patient in the emergency room and intensive care unit.

Throughout the clinical course, Tom met regularly with the clinical teachers to discuss matters related to the course and student progress. As well, he met informally with clinical staff. Tom was struck by the remarks of both teachers and staff that it took the students a long time "to get up to speed" in the clinical sites. He also noted on the clinical evaluations that many students were hesitant about the technical equipment, had difficulty attaching meaning to signs of rapidly changing physiological status, and/or felt overwhelmed by the clinical situations.

Tom discussed the situation with Sandra Greenberg, a trusted friend and pediatric intensive care nursing specialist who was responsible for the course in children's health, which is prerequisite to Tom's course. She said that students reacted in a similar fashion when assigned to the pediatric units of the tertiary care teaching hospital where she does clinical teaching.

Sandra and Tom believed they must do everything possible to ensure that students completing the program are able to provide competent, hospital-based care in situations of high acuity. Together, they began to consider reshaping the undergraduate curriculum to emphasize enhanced knowledge and skill development related to tertiary-level care. For example, they talked about reconfiguring the family nursing courses to address care of ICU patients' families. They would like to see curriculum changes implemented in the next academic year so that successive classes will be "up to speed."

Knowing that they need the support of nursing faculty, Tom and Sandra tested their ideas with a few faculty whose class or clinical teaching is aligned with acute care nursing, as well as with other intensive care clinical nursing specialists. All were supportive of the idea of increasing the focus on acute and intensive care in the curriculum and most said they will do whatever possible to help. Filled with enthusiasm for their plan, Tom and Sandra arranged a meeting with the Undergraduate Program Chair, certain that their ideas would be welcomed.

Critique The reasons for the proposed curriculum revision were Tom's once-only experience in teaching the class and clinical courses about nursing of clients with complex needs, students' clinical performance evaluations, and comments from other acute-care teachers and clinical staff. As well, Tom and Sandra wanted to ensure that graduating students would be able to provide competent hospital-based care. They were enthusiastic about a curriculum revision, but lacked a sufficient database upon which to recommend a change from the current program.

Tom and Sandra needed to examine the curriculum philosophy and intent, review the original course goals, and determine the expected level of performance for graduating students. Was the course really meant to focus on intensive care and emergency situations? They also needed more concrete information about what it meant for students not to be "up to speed" on the units, and determine whether being "up to speed" is a reasonable expectation.

Tom and Sandra had the support of others with a similar clinical focus, but they had not yet explored their perspective with faculty whose teaching lies in the areas of family nursing, mental health nursing, or community health. They did not consider that the current curriculum represented the most recent judgment of faculty. Moreover, while still introducing a new curriculum, it is unlikely that most faculty will be interested in revamping it.

Lacking a strong rationale for a curriculum change, Tom and Sandra cannot expect their ideas to be warmly received nor acted upon. Rather, they would be wise to examine the curriculum documents and determine if their courses and expectations of students are congruent with the curriculum intent. As well, they should consider whether allegiance to their clinical specialties has overshadowed the broader perspective of nursing which is required in undergraduate education. Tom and Sandra have gained tentative support from faculty and clinical personnel with a vested interest in acute care nursing. However, without strong evidence of the need for change in the current program, they cannot expect widespread support.

Stonehill University School of Nursing

Dr. Sylvia Weathersmith is dean and professor of Stonehill University School of Nursing. Enrollment is 425 undergraduate students and 75 graduate students. The teaching staff comprise 25 full-time faculty (5 PhD, 20 masters-prepared) and 35 part-time faculty (15 masters-prepared, 20 baccalaureate). There has been no revision of the undergraduate curriculum for several years.

Dr. Weathersmith is an active member of the university administrators group, the community health administrators association, and of several other professional organizations. She keeps abreast of changes in health care as well as in nursing education, and enjoys excellent relationships with faculty members as well as with nursing and non-nursing colleagues.

Twenty-four percent of undergraduates failed the last NCLEX. This percentage, along with limited research and publication activity, unsatisfactory ratings of graduates by employers, and a nursing curriculum based solely on a behaviorist model, has led to concerns about the upcoming accreditation review.

Although faculty have attended workshops and conferences on new and evolving educational paradigms, they are generally comfortable with the present curriculum. Three full-time faculty are excited about a caring, humanistic-educative approach. Dr. Weathersmith has called faculty together for a special meeting to discuss possible revisions to the undergraduate curriculum. The discussion centers on the status of the BSN program, particularly the need for change, as evidenced by the NCLEX results.

Questions for Consideration and Analysis of the Stonehill University Case

1. What factors or influences would precipitate curriculum revision in the undergraduate program?
2. Who should be involved if the decision to revise the curriculum is agreed upon?
3. What would be a suitable timeframe in light of the reasons for curriculum revision?
4. How would Dr. Weathersmith assess whether the faculty members accept the need for curriculum revision?

Curriculum Development Activities for Consideration in Your Setting

The following questions are intended to stimulate your thinking about curriculum development in your setting.

1. Why is curriculum development necessary now? What is the evidence for believing we should proceed?
2. Do we have enough substantive information on which to base our decision to proceed?
3. How can we present evidence about the need for curriculum change so it is convincing to others?
4. How extensive do we believe curriculum development should be? Should it be a revision of the current curriculum or a completely new curriculum?
5. From whom do we need to gain support for the idea of curriculum development?
6. How do we gain support?
   - What are the advantages and disadvantages of approaching colleagues individually or collectively?
   - How will participation in the curriculum change process affect faculty members' other commitments?
7. In addition to the need for curriculum change, what else should we be prepared to discuss with the dean or director in a preliminary way?
8. Who should be involved in the curriculum development process?
9. What will the timeframe be?
10. What resources will we need to be successful? Are there funding sources to support these activities?
11. What potential risks are associated with not going forward at this time?
12. What other considerations should require thoughtful attention at this time?

References

Attridge, C.B. (1996). Factors confounding the development of innovative roles and practices. *Journal of Nursing Education, 35,* 406–412.

Bevis, E.O. (2000a). Illuminating the issues. In E.O. Bevis & J. Watson (Eds.), *Toward a caring curriculum. A new pedagogy for nursing* (pp. 13–35). Boston: Jones and Bartlett Publishers.

Bevis, E.O. (2000b). Practical decision making about curriculum. In E.O. Bevis & J. Watson (Eds.), *Toward a caring curriculum. A new pedagogy for nursing* (pp. 107–152). Boston: Jones and Bartlett Publishers.

Bevis, E.O., & Clayton, G. (1988). Needed: A new curriculum development design. *Nurse Educator, 13*(4), 14–18.

Bowen, M., Lyons, K.J., & Young, B.E. (2000). Nursing and health care reform: Implications for curriculum development. *Journal of Nursing Education, 39*(1), 27–33.

Carmon, M., Hauber, R.P., & Chase, L. (1992). From anxiety to action. Facilitating faculty development during curricular change. *Nursing and Health Care, 13,* 364–368.

Conley, V.C. (1973). *Curriculum and instruction in nursing,* Boston: Little Brown and Co.

Diekelmann, N. (1997). Creating a new pedagogy for nursing. *Journal of Nursing Education, 36*(4), 147–148.

Freeman, L.H., Voignier, R.R., & Scott, D.L. (2002). New curriculum for a new century: Beyond repackaging. *Journal of Nursing Education, 41*(1), 38–40.

Graubard, A. (2000). Editor's preface. In E.O. Bevis & J. Watson (Eds.), *Toward a caring curriculum. A new pedagogy for nursing* (pp. xiii). Sudbury, MA: Jones and Bartlett Publishers.

Heller, B.R., Oros, M.T., & Durney-Crowley, J. (2000). The future of nursing education. 10 trends to watch. *Nursing and Health Care Perspectives, 21*(1), 9–13.

Howell Adams, M., Sherrod, D.R., Forte, L., Barnett Lamon, C.A., Stover, L.M., Shaw, Morrison, R., & Barrett, J.C. (2001). Restructuring a curriculum to meet future health care needs. *Nurse Educator, 26*(1), 6–8.

Lindeman, C.A. (2000). The future of nursing education. *Journal of Nursing Education, 39*(1), 5–12.

Moccia, P. (1990). No sire. It's a revolution. *Journal of Nursing Education, 29*(7), 307–310.

Oermann, M.H. (1995). Anniversary update. The progress of nursing education. *Nurse Educator, 29*(1), 4–10.

Pesut, D.J. (1995). Anniversary update. The progress of nursing education. *Nurse Educator, 29*(1), 4–10.

Rentschler, D.D., & Spegman, A.D. (1996). Curriculum revolution: Realities of change. *Journal of Nursing Education, 35,* 389–393.

Rush, K.L., Ouellet, L.L., & Wasson, D. (1991). Faculty development: the essence of curriculum development. *Nurse Education Today, 11,* 121–126.

Tappan, R.M. (2001). *Nursing leadership and management; Concepts and practice.* (4th ed.). Philadelphia: F. A. Davis Company.

Thornton, R., & Chapman, H. (2000). Student voice in curriculum making. *Journal of Nursing Education, 39,* 124–132.

Watson, J. (2000a). A new paradigm of curriculum development. In E.O. Bevis & J. Watson (Eds.), *Toward a caring curriculum. A new pedagogy for nursing* (pp. 37–49). Boston: Jones and Bartlett Publishers.

Watson, J. (2000b). Transformative thinking. In E.O. Bevis & J. Watson (Eds.), *Toward a caring curriculum. A new pedagogy for nursing* (pp. 51–60). Boston: Jones and Bartlett Publishers.

CHAPTER 3

Organizing for Curriculum Development: The Practical Considerations

Chapter Overview

This chapter provides practical guidelines about the first steps of curriculum development that will be helpful for organizing the work ahead. Once a decision has been made to proceed with curriculum development, it is essential that the enterprise be organized in such a way that the work can be satisfactorily completed in a timely fashion. Matters such as leadership, committee structure, decision-making, concrete work plans, authorship and academic freedom, faculty development, and the acquisition of resources must be decided before the process of curriculum development can begin. Remember, there is no precise sequence for attending to these issues: in reality they are usually addressed concurrently and in an iterative fashion, with one idea influencing another. As well, agreements achieved about leadership, decision-making approaches, committee structure, and so forth are all subject to review and revision as curriculum development proceeds.

A discussion of activities associated with getting organized for curriculum development is followed by an introduction to faculty development as part of this initial organization. The synthesis activities that conclude the chapter include, first, a case study and critique to illustrate the foremost points of the chapter, followed by a second case for analysis. Included are questions to determine readiness to begin curriculum development.

Chapter Goals

- Overview factors important in organizing for curriculum development
- Consider methods to organize for curriculum development
- Identify activities involved when organizing for curriculum development
- Contemplate faculty development activities related to organizing for curriculum development

Organizing for Curriculum Development

Deciding on Leadership

Deciding on leadership is an important aspect of organizing for curriculum development. Questions to be answered are: what is leadership and what is involved in effective leadership? What style of leadership would be most effective? Who should be the leader and how should this person guide the process?

Few topics in the social sciences have attracted as much commentary, theory, and research as that of leaders and leadership. Schools of thought about leadership have been evolutionary, and there is an expanding body of knowledge on the subject. Progression has occurred from the great man theory, to trait or characteristics of leaders, to behavioral theory, and from a focus on the individual leader to leaders and followers, and to the situation and environment. The following summary of leadership may help potential curriculum leaders assess their aptitude for this role.

Leadership Leadership is the process of influencing people to accomplish goals or to move toward goal setting and achievement. It is generally conceived that any person can use the leadership process, that it can be learned, and that anyone can become a leader in primarily one of two ways. First, a leader can be informally chosen or formally elected by members of a group who recognize and accept the leader's influence to lead, and who view the leader as someone who is competent and trustworthy. This is referred to as *emergent leadership*. Secondly, a leader may be appointed or elected to the position by people external to the group. This is called *im-*

posed or *organizational leadership*. Imposed leaders may have difficulty being accepted by the group or receiving support because of lack of trust.

Effective Leadership   To lead successfully, leaders must possess knowledge, skills, and a caring and compassionate attitude, since leading is essentially about people (Yoder-Wise, 1995). Obviously, leadership roles in curriculum development are multiple, due to the numerous environments in which the work is conducted and the levels at which leaders must operate. In fact, 19 roles applicable to a curriculum leader have been identified: expert, instructor, trainer, retriever, referrer, linker, demonstrator, modeler, advocate, confronter, counselor, advisor, observer, data collector, analyzer, diagnoser, designer, manager, and evaluator (Havelock and Associates as cited in Wiles & Bondi, 1998).

Interrelated attributes for effective leaders include awareness of self and group members, advocacy for the group, and accountability for one's actions to self, group, profession, and superiors (Bernhard & Walsh, 1990). Five practices associated with exceptional leadership are:

- challenging the process by searching for opportunities, experimenting, and taking risks
- inspiring a shared vision by envisioning the future and enlisting the support of others
- enabling others to act by fostering collaboration and strengthening others
- modeling the way by setting an example and planning small successes
- encouraging the heart by recognizing contributions and celebrating accomplishments (Huber, 2000)

Three levels of leadership have also been identified: individual, in which leaders mentor, coach and motivate; group, where leaders build teams and resolve conflicts; and organizational, in which leaders build a culture (Huber, 2000). Three suggested skills needed for effective leadership are: diagnosing (understanding the situation); adapting (matching behaviors and resources to the situation); and communicating (advancing the [curriculum] process in ways that individuals can understand and accept) (Hersey, Blanchard, & Johnson, 1996).

Effective Leadership Styles   Leadership styles have been extensively studied since the time of Plato. Former classic works of leadership styles, namely *democratic, autocratic,* and *laissez-faire,* have been replaced with other approaches which conceptualize styles in terms of task (Cartwright & Zender, 1960); leader views of followers (McGregor, 1960; Blake & Mouton, 1964); variables of task structure and position power (Fiedler, 1967); and two- and three-dimensional models of effectiveness (Hersey et al., 1996). The current view is that one style is not necessarily better than another, as many factors impact on leaders and leadership styles (Goldenberg, 1990). Each has advantages and disadvantages, and styles vary according to the situation.

A focus on the relationship between leaders and followers has led to the identification of transactional and transformative leadership. *Transactional* leaders function within the existing organizational culture in a care-giving role, concern themselves with day-to-day operations, set goals expected of the group, and assign rewards in an exchange posture or bargain contract, for mutual benefit. Transactional leaders manage by exception, a technique found to be an essential component of effective leadership in some situations.

Transformational leaders motivate the group to perform to their full potential over time, by influencing a change in perceptions and by providing a sense of direction. These leaders use charisma, individualized consideration and intellectual satisfaction in the group, and engage with others so that they and the group members raise each other to higher levels of motivation and ethical decision-making. These leaders focus on collective purpose, mutual growth and development; they have a vision, and empower others to expend extra effort beyond performance expectations. They develop pride and satisfaction in the work, enthusiasm, team spirit, and a sense of accomplishment. This style is better suited to the work of professionals (Bass & Avolio, 1990), and would be most effective for curriculum leaders.

Current views of effective leadership have evolved from principles of quantum mechanics and reflect an intermingling of trait, behavior and contingency approaches (Sullivan & Decker, 2005). Some of these include the following leadership styles:

- *quantum,* based on chaos theory, involves facilitative leaders and equitably involved participants
- *charismatic,* based on personal characteristics and qualities, involves charming, persuasive leaders and affectionate, committed participants
- *shared,* based on empowerment principles, involves participative, transformational leaders and empowered, knowledgeable participants
- *servant,* based on desire to serve; involves serving-other leaders and evolving serving-other participants.

Appointing the Curriculum Leader

Most schools will have a formal leader for the curriculum development process. The curriculum leader might be the undergraduate Chair or another faculty member who is deemed to be appropriate. This individual could be appointed by the dean or director, or determined by faculty members. Typically, this will be an appointed position, since the inherent responsibilities will have implications for other aspects of the person's workload. Among the curriculum leader's specific responsibilities are to:

- ensure that curriculum development activities proceed in a timely fashion to meet agreed-upon deadlines
- negotiate with the school dean or director for adequate resources for curriculum development

- serve as an ex officio member of the Curriculum Committee (if not already a member)
- consult with subcommittees about their activities, as requested
- initiate discussion (and perhaps negotiate) with other departments about support courses
- liaise with the school dean or director, Advisory Committee, and the nursing community
- arrange for faculty development activities
- prepare reports and finalize documents for institutional approval of the curriculum
- assist in marketing the new or revised curriculum

The curriculum leader should be expert in curriculum matters, able to initiate and direct the curriculum process, familiar with the institution and the required approvals for the new or redesigned curriculum, skilled in effective group functioning, and able to use an effective style appropriate to the curriculum participants and situation. Although knowledgeable about the curriculum development process, substance and relevance of the work done, the curriculum leader does not have decision-making authority about the new curriculum. That authority rests with the director of the school and the faculty. However, the leader does have responsibility for ensuring that the curriculum is developed in a timely fashion, and this requires working effectively with members of all committees that are formed.

An alternative to selecting or appointing an internal leader is to seek direction from a curriculum consultant, who might be appointed for a short term. It is important to remember, however, that consultants should be chosen carefully according to their area of expertise related to curriculum development and to the needs of the faculty. Typically, external consultants are short-term adjuncts to curriculum development, rather than an integral part of the daily activities.

Deciding on Committee Structure

After agreement is reached about issues of leadership and decision-making for the curriculum task, getting organized involves considering which committees to form and determining their structure and functions. Committees are essential for developing a curriculum, not only because the work must be shared, but also because the discussion that occurs during meetings leads to agreement and acceptance of ideas.

Organizing for Committee Structure The key to successful curriculum development is a committee structure conducive to the task, yet amenable to modification if necessary. Activities of all committees and subcommittees ought to proceed in an organized fashion, be based on realistic expectations, and be supported by adequate resources. When structuring committees, important considerations are the purposes of the committee, tasks to be accomplished, methods of achieving the work, deadlines for completion, and membership. These are the *what, how, who,* and *when* aspects of the proposed committees.

The committee structure (number, purpose, and membership of committees) needs to be considered carefully so that it is facilitative of curriculum development. This requires attention to determining the best way to accomplish the curriculum development work and associated responsibilities (such as gaining community support), while ensuring inclusion of all faculty, interested students, and stakeholders. The types of committees that could be suitable and ideas about membership are presented below. Each committee or subcommittee should have a clear purpose; its accountability and deadlines defined.

Organizing also requires that the designated curriculum leader and members together establish strategies designed to achieve the task of curriculum development expeditiously. Policies, plans, and activities to accomplish the tasks, and the best way to use available human and material resources, must be agreed upon. Delegation of responsibility and authority to committees, groups, and individuals, tied together horizontally and vertically through facilitative relationships and information systems, will most likely be necessary to perform the activities (Koontz, O'Donnell, & Weihrich, 1986).

Within the committees, it is necessary to establish member roles, define tasks, schedule meetings, arrange for the recording of minutes, and do the work assigned within the specified timeline. Leadership for particular curriculum development activities may be temporary, as leaders could be appointed, elected, or rotated, and because subcommittees will disband when their work is completed. Membership on curriculum committees is usually based on interest, expertise, broad understanding of the program, school, and institution, as well as knowledge of teaching and learning. Collectively, curriculum participants should be familiar with the following: nursing education, curriculum process, philosophies, health care issues, available resources, requirements for graduation, evaluation, approval and/or accreditation standards, and licensing requirements.

Types of Committees   Undoubtedly, a workable committee structure includes a *Curriculum Committee* of dedicated, knowledgeable participants who will be responsible for the overall development of the proposed curriculum. Members of the Curriculum Committee will become members of subcommittees.

A possible committee structure could be one that allows all members to function as a *Total Faculty Group*, which develops and approves all curriculum proposals. This type of structure can be effective in a small school of nursing. However, in most schools, such a structure could slow curriculum development and therefore, it is more usual for the Total Faculty Group to come together to discuss, and approve the work of subcommittees. Use of a Total Faculty Group at critical points in curriculum development can promote faculty 'buy-in.'

The use of *subcommittees* or *task forces (ad hoc committees)* within the Curriculum Committee is another structure to consider. These facilitate optimal participation of all people involved in curriculum development. Discrete tasks such as collecting contextual data, formulating the philosophical approaches, writing curriculum goals, and so forth are given to the subcommittees. These small groups enable each participant to contribute and critique the work accomplished. They are transitory, task-oriented, and their dissolution is natural when the work is done. Usually, task forces do short term, small tasks, whereas subcommittees have the total ongoing responsibility of developing their portion of the curriculum and reporting back to the Curriculum Committee and the Total Faculty Group. Like subcommittees, task groups provide feedback and generate more than one alternative for every phase of their task. Each task force or subcommittee should set its own rules, announce plans, provide information, make conflicts explicit and legitimate, identify high investment areas and risks, incorporate changes and acceptable alternatives, agree to respond to each other's contributions, suggest ways to respond to deadlocked issues, and offer tentative or provisional decisions (Bevis, 1989).

It is important to remember that views of stakeholders and curriculum planners are to be obtained while small group members are working on specific tasks. This can be done by inviting them to become members or to attend selected committee or task force meetings; by interviews with faculty members; through survey tools for reactions to issues and ideas; and by Total Faculty Group meetings, with materials sent out beforehand for review. Perspectives of the total student body (in addition to student representation on committees) can be obtained in a similar manner.

In addition to subcommittees with responsibility for particular aspects of curriculum development, Bevis (1989) recommends the formation of a *Critique Committee* to review and comment on particular curriculum elements. A subcommittee such as this can ask questions, suggest clarification or expansion of some points, examine incongruencies, suggest revision, and provide feedback, thereby adding validity to the work. Whether or not a critique committee is formed, it is essential that all curriculum development participants be kept informed and have opportunities to provide input into subcommittees' work on an ongoing basis.

The school might also enlist the help of an *Advisory Committee*, made up of members from the academic and professional communities as well as consumers. These persons could be enlisted to serve on task forces or subcommittees. Advisory bodies are a useful source of information as well as a public relations mechanism to foster understanding and promotion of the curriculum.

Finally, a *Steering Committee* could be formed. This occurs most frequently when a curriculum is being planned and implemented by more than one institution. The committee membership can be comprised of senior administrators of the institutions, directors of the nursing program(s), and the curriculum chair(s). The number and organizational position of members from the involved institutions are usually equal. The Steering Committee might:

- offer direction to the joint curriculum initiative
- ensure that plans are in accordance with institutional policies, or alternatively identify needed changes in policies
- plan for sharing of resources, if appropriate
- liaise with institutional governing bodies and external bodies (e.g., nursing regulatory or government) as necessary.

It is prudent to consider the inclusion of senior administrators, not only on the Advisory and Steering Committees, but on subcommittees as well. This will keep them apprised of curriculum developments and lessen the possibility of surprises and potential vetoes (Bevis, 1989).

Whatever committee structure is used, it is important to remember that the potential for success in curriculum development is directly related to the degree of participation of stakeholders. The greater the participation, the greater the success that will result (Torres & Stanton, 1982).

Recordkeeping Meeting minutes are essential, and these should be up-to-date and complete. Copies of working papers, documents, and minutes used or developed by the committee members should be dated and retained. It is important to inventory what has been done and what is usable. These materials are a history of the development of the curriculum, the story of how the curriculum unfolds and of how ideas evolve from abstractions to operational activities (Torres & Stanton, 1982).

Attached to the formal meeting minutes should be any substantive discussion or decisions that have occurred via email between meetings. Much work is done between meetings, of course, and the email discussion among group members can easily be retained as part of the "paper trail" of the group's thinking and decisions. To a large extent, the emails form the minutes.

An alternative to email can be the establishment of a computer conference site for curriculum discussion. A secure, accessible, online space allows for multiple, asynchronous, threaded discussions. The use of such a program will allow those involved in curriculum development to keep abreast of the work of all subcommittees. Most importantly, messages are dated and can be reviewed and printed to accompany or serve as minutes.

Determining Decision-making Approaches

An important activity in the development of curriculum is decision-making. It is an organizational element inherent in curriculum change (Conley, 1973), as decisions must be agreed upon in order to complete the curriculum. Curriculum developers, therefore, must concur about which decision-making processes would be acceptable to them.

Decision-making A decision is a choice among alternatives, while decision-making is more complex, as it involves the act of choosing, and converting information into action. It is a systematic process that begins with a need or problem, and ends when an evaluation of the choice is completed (Bernhard & Walsh, 1990; Grainger, 1990). Moreover, decision-making differs from problem solving in that it is influenced by emotions and intuition, is purposeful and goal-oriented, involves a choice among options, and may not always start with a problem (Huber, 2000).

Decision-making might also be the "result of opportunities, challenges, or leadership initiatives" (Huber, 2000, p. 378). It implies responsibility, and anticipation of consequences. Decision-making is considered to be the essence of leadership, and making decisions could be the most important aspect of a job, the most difficult, and the riskiest. Good decisions usually lead to attainment of goals, whereas bad decisions can impede progress, waste resources, cause harm or damage, and ultimately affect careers. Huber offers some core elements of decision-making:

- identifying a problem, issue or situation
- establishing criteria for evaluating potential solutions
- searching for alternative solutions or actions
- evaluating the alternatives
- choosing specific alternatives (Huber, 2000)

Some decision-making techniques are outlined in Table 3.1.

TABLE 3.1   DECISION-MAKING TECHNIQUES

- trial and error
- pilot project
- problem critique: technique in which problem is outlined, facts determined, and potential solutions proposed
- creativity techniques: brainstorming, delphi process, and nominal group
- decision tree or critical pathways
- fish-bone (or cause and effect chart)
- group problem solving and decision-making
- cost-benefit analysis
- worst case scenario

[Data from Huber, D. (2000). *Leadership and nursing care management.* (2nd ed.). Philadelphia: W. B. Saunders, pp. 384–387].

Decision-making Styles Not only is decision-making thought of as a process with identifiable steps, there are various decision-making styles, types (models), and strategies. Decision styles, as with leadership, range from *authoritarian* or *autocratic*, in which the leader makes the decision alone; *consultative*, *collective* or *participative*, where the leader seeks input before making the final decision; *facilitative*, in which the leader and group combined reach a shared decision; and *delegative*, where only the group makes the decision and the leader gives up control over the decision (Hersey, Blanchard, & Johnson, 1996).

Types of decisions described by Bernhard and Walsh (1990) are twofold: *satisficing*, which implies choosing any solution that will satisfy or minimally meet the desired goals; and *optimizing*, which involves comparing all possible solutions against the goals and choosing the one that best meets them. Satisficing decisions are easier to make as the decision-maker chooses the first and quickest solution for solving the problem, while sacrificing a fuller analysis of the situation. The speed of the decision might even inspire support from the group. In order to find the best solution, with the potential for effectiveness and acceptability by the group, an optimizing solution would be the logical choice (Bernhard & Walsh).

Optimal Curriculum Decisions Curriculum design and construction can never become a matter of routine or formula. Curriculum development must rely on decisions determined by a variety of ideas, imagination, facts, theories, creativity, and even prejudices. Furthermore, curriculum decision-making is complicated as it involves people who have various levels of curriculum expertise, vested interests, private hopes and dreams, different ideas and emotions, and the desire to give the best possible education for students (Bevis, 2000).

Decisions about curriculum should not be constrained by rules or rigid formulae, but rather be guided by desired curriculum goals, acceptability by the group, effective strategies, and internal and external contextual factors. (Chapter 5 will address data-gathering about contextual factors). Decision-makers should acknowledge that previous decisions influence each new or subsequent decision and that new decisions may lead to a reconsideration of previous choices. Optimal decision-making, therefore, is an iterative, dynamic, and interactive process grounded in contextual reality.

Establishing a Work Plan

When engaged in curriculum work, participants will have to redirect time and energy from other activities into curriculum development. Resources may have to be shifted from one committee to another. Assigning time to work on the curriculum during summer or release time, a usual practice, is not always effective, as communications break down and commitment to the developing curriculum is substantially reduced.

Curriculum development is a slow process, the period of time for completion usually based on the frequency of meetings. It cannot be effective if crisis-oriented approaches are used. A written, realistic timetable to guide the activities of the group is important, as it places the activity in the context of its priority and the group's commitment to the goals. It will help to maintain participant interest, and support the expectation that a new or revised curriculum will be accomplished. Too short a time could be self-defeating, and viewed as a lack of regard for members' time and other responsibilities.

A productive approach is one that provides regular meetings at which participants can assess decisions step-by-step and plan for the next activity by studying and creating new ideas (Torres & Stanton, 1982). If there are enough committed and qualified committee members who have expertise or who seek assistance, and who also meet on a regular basis, the goal of a developed curriculum will be achieved in a timely manner. It is neither practical nor productive to spend an extensive period of time on any one component of the curriculum. Despite the discomfort that may accompany decisions that are not firmly fixed, the group should move on to completion. As the work progresses through subsequent meetings, final decisions can be accomplished.

A prerequisite for undertaking a project as large as curriculum development is establishing a work plan. Major elements of the curriculum development process must be identified and a timeline specified, responsibility assigned for activities, procedures determined for recording meeting minutes and decisions, and the work shared. Initial decisions may need to be reviewed as the work progresses and circumstances not apparent at the outset become evident. The creation of a work plan will bring definition to the curriculum development process.

Critical Path The critical path is a blueprint for action, specifying the steps to be completed, the deadlines, and the individuals or committees responsible for each phase of the curriculum development process. It will provide a concrete means to assess whether the curriculum is being developed at a pace that will ensure implementation by the target date. Dates of key meetings and reporting intervals (Smith, 1999) can be included as part of the critical path. Although revisions may become necessary, the critical path explicates the work to be done and the timeframe in which it must be completed. Importantly, a detailed critical path is the rationale for requesting resources.

Agreeing on deadlines for the major milestones of curriculum development is the first step in the creation of a critical path. Typically, the initial decision is to identify the implementation date of the first courses, by placing this first on the critical path. This highlights or gives preeminence to the start date for the new or revised curriculum. After deciding when the curriculum is to begin, determine the total amount of time available to finalize it by calculating back to the date the educational institution must approve the curriculum design. Identifying major activities that must occur before final approval, and the associated deadlines for each, is the next step. It is helpful to note which individual or committee will have responsibility for each aspect of the process, as well as the approval procedures necessary throughout curriculum development. As the process evolves, committees will find it helpful to develop their own critical paths.

Table 3.2 provides an example of a critical path, beginning with the implementation date of the curriculum and working backward in time to when the curriculum development

TABLE 3.2   EXAMPLE OF A CRITICAL PATH FOR CURRICULUM DEVELOPMENT

Activities to be Completed	Deadline (Time from Start Date)	Individual or Group Responsible
Implement 1st year of new curriculum	36 months	School Director
Prepare detailed syllabi of 1st year courses	33 months	Course professors
Interpret curriculum to clinical agencies, professional bodies	30 months	Curriculum leader Curriculum committee
Prepare web site, recruitment and marketing materials	24 months	Curriculum leader Curriculum committee Marketing consultant Web designer
Prepare necessary documents for approval of curriculum by university governing body	24 months	Curriculum leader School Director
Present curriculum to Advisory Body	24 months	Curriculum leader
Prepare and present motions for curriculum approval by Total Faculty Group	24 months	Curriculum leader
Present curriculum to Steering Committee	23 months	Curriculum leader
Finalize curriculum design and policies	22 months	Total Faculty Group
Refine and negotiate courses and policies	20 months	Curriculum Committee Designated subcommittees
Present program policies to Curriculum Committee	18 months	Program policy subcommittee
Present course descriptions, goals, and major content areas to Curriculum Committee	18 months	Course development teams
Establish course development teams	13 months	Curriculum Committee
Finalize curriculum matrix	13 months	Total Faculty Group
Negotiate support courses	12 months	Curriculum leader

Activities to be Completed	Deadline (Time from Start Date)	Individual or Group Responsible
Develop curriculum matrix with nursing and non-nursing courses	10 months	Curriculum Committee
Finalize program philosophical approaches and goals	8 months	Total Faculty Group
Present draft program goals to Curriculum Committee	6 months	Goals subcommittee
Present draft philosophical approaches to Curriculum Committee	6 months	Philosophical approaches subcommittee
Agree on general direction of curriculum philosophical approaches, goals, concepts, and potential curriculum design	4 months	Total Faculty Group
Present synthesis of contextual data	4 months	Data collection subcommittee
Collect contextual data	3 months	Data collection subcommittee
Establish subcommittees and task forces	Immediately	Curriculum Committee
Initiate faculty development	Immediately and ongoing	Curriculum leader
Identify major steps of curriculum development process and create critical path	Immediately	Curriculum Committee
Form Advisory Committee	Immediately	School Director Curriculum leader
Form Steering Committee	Immediately	School Director, and/or Nominations and Elections Committee
Appoint Curriculum leader	Immediately	School Director with faculty input

process actually begins. A three-year period for the development of a typical four-year undergraduate program is presented in consideration of the time needed for the change process among faculty (Mawn & Reece, 2000), various levels of approval that may exist in some institutions, and realities of faculty members' other responsibilities. Once the reverse ordering is completed, the chart can be rotated so that it starts with the most immediate activities and ends with curriculum implementation. This is the critical path. Alternately a Gantt chart could be devised. The advantage of the Gantt chart is that it illustrates the duration of activities. A Gantt chart to match Table 3.2 is presented in Table 3.3.

Many other activities and meetings could be added to the critical path. For example, meetings of the Total Faculty Group and the Curriculum Committee might be included, as well as regular meetings with the school director. It is important to find a comfortable balance such that the critical path can specify the major work to be done without being overly detailed. Committees or individuals can develop other critical paths to ensure that their work will be completed to match the major deadlines.

Approaches to Sharing the Work   Inherent in all group work is the need to determine how activities will be completed. Who will do what, and to what standard? This is partly accomplished by decisions about committee structures. Yet, within each committee, the matter of how to share the work will arise, and the approach is unlikely to be identical in each committee and subcommittee. In some, all members may prefer to work together as much as possible, so ideas are explored and consensus is achieved before much writing is done. For others, there may be a desire to divide tasks among individuals or dyads, and then bring back draft work to the group for discussion, revision, and consensus. Likely, some combination of these approaches will be agreed to, depending on the nature of the task and the imminence of deadlines. Although it is beyond the scope of this book to describe all aspects of successful group functioning, some elements are worthy of review when considering how the work of curriculum development can be accomplished.

- Agree on the goals to be achieved. This includes not only the task to be completed, but the deadline for completion and the standard of the work.
- Obtain commitment from each of the members to achieve the goal.
- Identify how much time each member can give to the task.
- Discuss how the group will work together.
- Consider the value of preparing a critical path for the group's work.
- Recognize that not all workgroups will become cohesive teams, whose synergy is intrinsically motivating (Wylie & Smith, 1999).

Schedule of Meetings   Developing a schedule of meetings for committees and task forces will both expedite the work of curriculum development and keep the groups on track for

TABLE 3.3   GANTT CHART FOR CURRICULUM DEVELOPMENT

Task/Activity	Accountability	Time in Months From Start Date													
		0	1	2	3	4	5	6	7	8	9	10	11	12	13
Appoint Curriculum Leader	School Director	▨													
Form Steering Committee and Advisory Body	School Director and Curriculum leader	▨													
Identify major steps; create critical path; establish subcommittees	Curriculum Committee	▨													
Plan, implement faculty development	Curriculum leader	▨	▨	▨	▨	▨	▨	▨	▨	▨	▨	▨	▨	▨	▨
Collect and synthesize contextual data and present to Curriculum Committee	Data collection subcommittee			▨	▨										
Agree on general directions of curriculum philosophical approaches, goals, and major foci	Total Faculty Group			▨	▨										
Prepare draft philosophical approaches and present to Curriculum Committee	Philosophical approaches subcommittee		▨	▨	▨	▨	▨	▨							

continues

TABLE 3.3   CONTINUED

Task/Activity	Accountability	Time in Months From Start Date													
		0	1	2	3	4	5	6	7	8	9	10	11	12	13
Finalize philosophical approaches and goals	Total Faculty Group									▨					
Develop curriculum matrix	Curriculum Committee										▨	▨			
Negotiate support courses	Curriculum leader												▨	▨	
Finalize curriculum matrix	Total Faculty Group														▨
Establish course development teams	Curriculum Committee														▨

Task/Activity	Accountability	14	15	16	17	18	19	20	21	22	23	24	30	33	36
Plan, implement faculty development	Curriculum leader	X	X	X	X	X	X	X	X	X	X	X	X	X	X
Prepare course goals, descriptions and major content areas and present to Curriculum Committee	Course development teams	X	X	X	X	X									
Prepare program policies and present to Curriculum Committee	Policy subcommittee	X	X	X	X	X									
Refine & negotiate about courses and policies	Curriculum Committee and subcommittee					X	X	X							
Finalize curriculum design and policies	Total faculty group								X	X					
Present curriculum to Steering Committee	Curriculum leader										X				
Present curriculum to Advisory Body	Curriculum leader											X			
Prepare documents for curriculum approval by governing body	Curriculum leader											X	X	X	X

continues

TABLE 3.3   CONTINUED

Task/Activity	Accountability	Time in Months From Start Date													
		14	15	16	17	18	19	20	21	22	23	24	30	33	36
Prepare web site, recruiting and marketing materials	Curriculum leader, Curriculum Committee, consultants									▨	▨	▨			
Interpret curriculum to clinical agencies, professional bodies	Curriculum Committee											▨	▨	▨	▨
Prepare detailed syllabi for first courses	Course professors											▨	▨		
Implement curriculum	School Director														▨

completion of their tasks. These can be included in the critical path, or a separate listing of meeting dates can be prepared to coincide with the critical path. In either case, early development of a meeting schedule with a notation about the major task to be achieved will help to ensure that curriculum developers reserve the time for meetings and that curriculum work proceeds in a timely fashion.

Securing Resources

As the overall plan for curriculum development is shaped, the necessary resources will become apparent. Concrete requests for resources should be made. The requests could include release time from teaching for key curriculum developers; a specific budget for data collection activities, faculty development, or curriculum consultation; and secretarial support. Although alterations in work assignments may be subject to collective agreements, they are worthy of exploration, since it is primarily the faculty who must develop, accept, and implement the curriculum.

Discussing the Relationship of Curriculum Development to Academic Freedom

Academic freedom is "the free search for truth and its free exposition" (American Association of University Professors [AAUP, n.d.]). This includes freedom in teaching, research, publication, and criticism of the institution. However, "academic freedom is a qualified right; . . . a privilege enjoyed in consequence of incumbency in . . . an academic role and it is enjoyed conditionally in conformity with certain obligations to the academic institution and its rules and standards" (Shils, 1993, p. 189).

Larson (1997) suggests that faculty sometimes perceive academic freedom as giving each faculty member the right to plan courses independently, without attention to how these conform to the entire curriculum. She contends that this is not realistic nor should it be supported. Faculty are granted freedom in the classroom in discussing their subject (AAUP, n.d.; Canadian Association of University Teachers, 1979); yet teaching must be undertaken "with due respect to what is thought by qualified colleagues" (Shils, 1993, p. 190).

There must be unity and progression within professional curricula. Therefore, creating courses in isolation from one another and without reference to agreed-upon philosophical approaches and curriculum goals, is neither acceptable nor sound. Curriculum development, however, should not be so constrained that creativity, pedagogical preferences, and expertise of faculty are stifled. There should be a balance between faculty autonomy and curriculum intent. A frank discussion among faculty and the school leader would ensure resolution of the latitude possible within courses.

Contributing to curriculum development by all faculty is essential for a successful outcome. Because this requirement may compete with other scholarly activities, such as research, some faculty may feel their academic freedom is restricted. If this is the case, open discussion about academic rights and responsibilities is warranted, and thought should be given to adjustments in work assignments of some faculty.

Discussing Potential for Publication and Authorship

The possibility of publication arising from the curriculum development process should be discussed and agreed to in advance. Dialogue about this must occur early, since many expository and research articles could be generated as part of curriculum development.

Publications about the curriculum development process itself are important to consider. There may be aspects of the process that are unique, or insights attained that are worthy of sharing through journal articles. Often the 'lessons learned' are relevant to curriculum developers in other settings.

If it is decided that there are some researchable questions or other new knowledge to add to the body of curriculum development scholarship, the topic of authorship should be addressed. Many issues should be resolved early. For example, will one person or a team be responsible for writing proposals and articles? How will contributors be acknowledged in publications? Will primary authorship rotate among faculty and be dependent on who takes the leadership role in specific publications? Perhaps there are faculty on the curriculum development team who would thrive on being involved in research and writing, and these could be an added incentive for their participation in curriculum development.

Faculty Development

Faculty development is foundational to the creation and implementation of a curriculum that reflects a new perspective and is true to the espoused philosophical approaches. It is paramount that faculty move from established styles of thinking and interacting to methods that reflect the new vision. Therefore, faculty development must be preeminent throughout the curriculum development process.

Faculty development is a joint obligation of individual faculty, groups of faculty, and the school leader. Finke (2005) asserts that faculty development for the teaching role should include attention to competencies associated with curriculum and course development. These include knowledge of the content area; writing learning objectives; developing learning activities; selecting and presenting learning experiences; using appropriate teaching-learning theories in classroom and clinical settings; specifying expectations; providing feedback; facilitating development of critical thinking skills; using information technologies; and evaluating learning. These are essential skills for teachers and are prerequisite to curriculum development, but are not in themselves sufficient for curriculum development.

Faculty development has been described as the "essence of curriculum development" (Rush, Ouellet, & Wasson, 1991). Indeed, attention has been given to developing faculty to teach and to evaluate student learning in changed curricula (Bevis, 2000; Marcus, 1997; Rush, Ouellet, & Wasson; Torres & Stanton, 1982). However, faculty development about the curriculum development process itself is rarely addressed, perhaps because of an unexamined assumption that teachers implicitly know how to develop curricula, or perhaps because curriculum development activities have traditionally received little (if any) credit toward promotion and tenure decisions.

A significant curriculum revision or the development of a new curriculum will require faculty to look beyond their own clinical specialties and courses. They need to consider which philosophical approaches and concepts should underpin the curriculum, and what the curriculum goals, subject matter, and methods to achieve the goals should be. As well, they must examine how all aspects of a curriculum interact, and the best course configuration. To develop a unified curriculum in a timely fashion, faculty and other stakeholders might require assistance with the curriculum development process itself, as well as with curriculum implementation. Accordingly, faculty development must occur in tandem with curriculum development. Chapter 4 presents a description of faculty development, and each subsequent chapter includes ideas for faculty development related specifically to the chapter content.

Faculty Development Related to Organizing for Curriculum Development Once a decision has been made to proceed with curriculum development, it is worthwhile to have a faculty development session about the curriculum development process itself. Specifically, a summary of the entire process will help novices appreciate that curriculum development is an iterative process, replete with concurrent and recurrent subprocesses. However, to ensure that faculty do not feel overwhelmed, it is wise to identify the concrete tasks that ensure timely completion of the work. The goal is for faculty to comprehend the process and believe that it is manageable. Therefore, an overview of the logistics of getting organized is essential. Importantly, faculty development could also address the topic of leadership, since many faculty members assume leadership roles on various subcommittees or task forces involved in curriculum development.

Chapter Summary

Getting organized for curriculum development activities comprises attention to both the processes of working together and the logistics of getting the work done. Effective leadership and decision-making procedures are of paramount importance. Determining committee structures and establishing a work plan provide a concrete basis for progress. Inclusion of people beyond the nursing faculty will assist with completion of the work and broaden the perspectives of nursing faculty, and ultimately, the curriculum. Attention should be given to issues of academic freedom and publication possibilities at the outset, since these are directly relevant to the careers of nursing faculty. Finally, it is essential to secure the necessary resources to carry out the plans. Faculty development is integral to all these activities.

Synthesis Activities

Two cases are presented for review and discussion. The first is critiqued to identify the key elements of organizing for curriculum development. Read the case carefully and analyze Dr. Garcia's activities. Consider the analysis and propose additional or alternative ideas. The second is followed by questions to guide your critique. Finally, questions are presented about organizing for curriculum development.

Middlemount University School of Nursing

The Undergraduate Chair of Middlemount University, Dr. Simon Garcia, has gained support from a majority of faculty and the nursing school director to initiate the development of a new curriculum. This will be Dr. Garcia's first experience with such a large educational undertaking and he is eager to ensure that the process goes smoothly and quickly. A "take-charge" kind of person, Dr. Garcia immediately develops a critical path so the new curriculum can be implemented in 18 months. Knowing the skills of the faculty, Dr. Garcia begins to identify which faculty will be best suited for which activities. He consults with a few of the key faculty about how the curriculum development process might unfold. He then calls a meeting of all faculty who will be expected to participate in curriculum development to describe his plans to them.

Critique In his enthusiasm, Dr. Garcia has mistakenly taken on the roles of the curriculum leader and Curriculum Committee. Although it is reasonable that the undergraduate chair would have a key role, Dr. Garcia may not be the preferred leader of the group. The faculty may appreciate his "take charge" approach, but it would be wise to confirm the leadership with those who will be involved and with the school director. Since he does not have experience in such a large curriculum endeavor, Dr. Garcia may not be the best overall leader. His development of a critical path is premature, although it may serve as a model for one that is later developed by the Curriculum Committee. It is possible that the group will ask Dr. Garcia to formulate a draft critical path.

Dr. Garcia's motivation will be an important asset to the curriculum development process. However, he would be wise to ensure that his colleagues have full opportunity to participate in decisions about the process and extent of their involvement, congruent with expectations within the School. He needs to accept that many faculty will make only a tentative commitment to engage in curriculum work, not fully accepting responsibility for curriculum development until they are assured that the necessary resources have been secured. Moreover, some faculty may be unwilling to agree to participate in curriculum development simply because they are unsure of what the process involves.

Dr. Garcia could call a faculty meeting to report that there is support among faculty and from the school director for curriculum development. Together, they could then engage in the discussion that needs to precede the beginning of curriculum activities, that is, discussion about leadership, committee structures, decision-making processes, publication, faculty development, etc. Then, the critical path can be established. Concurrently, some initial faculty development could begin. Finally, once Dr. Garcia is sure about the extent to which individual faculty are willing to participate, he can return to the school director to secure the necessary resources.

Montag College Department of Nursing

Montag Community College (an associate degree-granting college) is located in a medium-sized metropolitan city of approximately 350,000 inhabitants. Health facilities include four hospitals as well as a visiting nurse service (which coordinates all community-based health care, except medical care) and several drop-in clinics. The College provides business, technology and health science programs to approximately 5000 postsecondary students. Among the programs is a 2-year, associate-degree nursing (ADN) program. Parkerville University is also located in the city and offers a 4-year baccalaureate program.

In addition to offering the 2-year ADN program, Montag College has entered into a partnership with Parkerville University to offer the first two years of the BSN program. Parkerville will offer the third and fourth years. There is agreement to develop a new curriculum together. Participants from both institutions and the health community are organizing to develop the new BSN curriculum.

Questions for Consideration and Analysis of the Montag College Case

1. What factors should be considered when deciding on leadership for curriculum development? What should be included in a faculty development program to prepare potential leaders? How might a leader be selected or appointed? Who should the leader be?

2. Identify factors that the curriculum developers should consider when embarking on the curriculum project.

3. What committees could be struck in order to facilitate curriculum development? What purposes would they serve? How should committee members be selected or appointed? Who should the members be?

4. What decision-making approaches would be effective for the curriculum developers?

5. Design a practical work plan for developing the curriculum.

6. What potential is there for publication arising from curriculum development? How might faculty determine authorship?

Curriculum Development Activities for Consideration in Your Setting

The following questions might stimulate thinking about organizing for curriculum development in your setting.

1. What qualities are important in a leader? What qualities could be important to faculty colleagues?

2. What approaches to decision-making do faculty most commonly use? How effective are they in achieving goals? Should we consider alternate approaches?

3. What kind of committee structure(s) for curriculum development might be most efficient and successful in our situation? Who should participate?

4. When do we want to implement the new curriculum? What is the best way to develop a critical path, and who will assume responsibility for developing it? What implications will curriculum development have for current faculty?

5. What are faculty's thoughts about academic freedom and the desire for publication?

6. Are sources of funding to support curriculum development available?

7. How is faculty development received in our situation? What strategies have been most effective in moving the group forward? How can we plan the faculty development activities we need now?

8. What types of resources to support curriculum development should be discussed with the administrator?

References

American Association of University Professors. (n.d.). 1940 Statement of Principles on Academic Freedom and Tenure with 1970 Interpretive Comments. Retrieved December 19, 2003 from *http://www.aaup.org/statements/Redbook/1940stat.htm.*

Bass, B., & Avolio, B. (1990). *Transformational leadership development: Manual for the multifactor leadership questionnaire.* Palo Alto, CA: Consulting Psychology Press.

Bernhard, L.A., & Walsh, M. (1990). *Leadership. The key to the professionalization of nursing.* (2nd ed.). St. Louis: C.V. Mosby.

Bevis, E.O. (1989). *Curriculum building in nursing. A process.* (3rd ed.). New York: National League for Nursing.

Bevis, E.O. (2000). Clusters of influence for practical decision-making about curriculum. In E.O. Bevis and J. Watson (Eds.), *Toward a caring curriculum: A new pedagogy for nursing.* (pp. 107–152). Boston: Jones and Bartlett Publishers.

Blake, R., & Mouton, J. (1964). *The managerial grid.* Houston, TX: Gulf Publishing.

Canadian Association of University Teachers. (1979). *CAUT Handbook.* Ottawa: Author.

Cartwright, D., & Zender, A. (Eds.). (1960). *Group dynamics: Research and theory.* (2nd ed.). Evanston, IL: Row, Paterson & Co.

Conley, V. (1973). *Curriculum and instruction in nursing.* Boston: Little Brown & Co.

Fiedler, F. (1967). *A theory of leadership effectiveness.* New York: McGraw-Hill.

Finke, L.M. (2005). Teaching in nursing: The faculty role. In D. M. Billings & J.A. Halstead (Eds.), *Teaching in Nursing: A Guide for Faculty.* (2nd ed.). (pp. 3–20). St. Louis: Elsevier Saunders.

Goldenberg, D. (1990). Nursing education leadership, effect of situational and constraint variables on leadership style. *Journal of Advanced Nursing, 15,* 1326–1334.

Grainger, D. (1990). Making better decisions. *American Journal of Nursing Education, 90*(6), 15–16.

Hersey, P., Blanchard, K.H., & Johnson, D.E. (1996). *Management of organizational behavior. Utilizing human resources.* (7th ed.). Upper Saddle River, N.J.: Prentice-Hall.

Huber, D. (2000). *Leadership and nursing care management.* (2nd ed.). Philadelphia: W.B. Saunders.

Koontz, H., O'Donnell, C., & Weihrich, J. (1986). *Essentials of management.* (4th ed.). New York: McGraw-Hill.

Larson, E. (1997). Academic freedom amidst competing demands. *Journal of Professional Nursing, 13*(4), 211–216.

Marcus, M.T. (1997). Faculty development and curricular change: A process and outcomes model for substance abuse education. *Journal of Professional Nursing, 13,* 168–177.

Mawn, B., & Reece, S.M. (2000). Reconfiguring a curriculum for the new millennium: The process of change. *Journal of Nursing Education, 39*(3), 101–108.

McGregor, D. (1960). *The human side of enterprise.* New York: McGraw-Hill.

Rush, K.L., Ouellet, L.L., & Wasson, D. (1991). Faculty development: The essence of curriculum development. *Nurse Education Today, 11,* 121–126.

Shils, E. (1993). Do we still need academic freedom? *The American Scholar, 62,* 187–207.

Smith, D. L. (1999). Project management. In J.M. Hibberd & D.L. Smith (Eds.). *Nursing management in Canada.* (2nd ed.). (pp. 471–485). Toronto: W. B. Saunders Canada.

Sullivan, E.J., & Decker, P. J. (2005). *Effective leadership and management in nursing.* (6th ed.). Upper Saddle River, N.J.: Pearson Prentice Hall.

Torres, G., & Stanton, M. (1982). *Curriculum process in nursing: A guide to curriculum development.* Englewood Cliffs, N.J.: Prentice-Hall.

Wiles, J., & Bondi, J. (1998). *Curriculum development: A guide to practice.* (5th ed.). Upper Saddle River, N.J.: Merrill, an imprint of Prentice Hall.

Wylie, D., & Smith, D.L. (1999). Leading and participating in workgroups and teams. In J. M. Hibberd & D.L. Smith (Eds.), *Nursing management in Canada.* (2nd ed.). (pp. 195–218). Toronto: W. B. Saunders Canada.

Yoder-Wise, P.S. (1995). *Leading and managing in nursing.* St. Louis: Mosby Year Book.

CHAPTER 4

Faculty Development and Change for Curriculum Development

Chapter Overview

This chapter addresses ideas about faculty development, an essential component of curriculum development activities. Although curriculum development is inherently a faculty development activity, ongoing planned faculty growth and evolution are also necessary to bring a new curriculum to fruition. In this chapter, attention is given to the meaning of, need for, and goals of faculty development, followed by a description of some useful activities to implement. The first section of the chapter concludes with a statement on faculty development related to curriculum development. Change theories are presented next, with application to faculty development for curriculum development. Then, strategies to support faculty during curriculum change, and ideas for responding to resistance to change, are offered. Synthesis activities include a case study and critique to exemplify important ideas, a second case for analysis, and questions to guide faculty development.

Chapter Goals

- Consider the need for faculty development as part of curriculum development
- Relate change and empowerment theories to faculty development

- Reflect on strategies to support faculty during change
- Ponder ideas for responding to resistance to faculty and curriculum development

Faculty Development for Curriculum Development

Faculty are the key players in the curriculum development and implementation processes: in decisions to be made, in committee work to be accomplished, and in teaching according to the tenets of a new or revised curriculum. Consequently, the success of curriculum change is largely dependent upon a knowledgeable and willing faculty.

Importantly, stakeholders such as clinicians, students, and administrators, who are part of the curriculum development process, should be included in faculty development activities. Participation in these learning opportunities will expand stakeholders' knowledge and skills about curriculum processes, and strengthen their connection with the school of nursing.

What Is Meant by 'Faculty Development'?

Faculty development can be conceived of as "the theory and practice of facilitating improved faculty performance in a variety of domains" (Halliburton, Marincovich, & Svinicki, 1988, p. 291). Traditionally, these domains have been personal and professional development, instructional development, and organizational development. Faculty development for curriculum development has not usually been included.

With a more specific focus on nurse educators, faculty development is defined as a "resocialization for faculty into educative processes that are liberating for both the educator and student" (Rush, Ouellet, & Wasson, 1991, p. 123). However, faculty development related to curriculum change is more extensive. It addresses all aspects of the curriculum development process, as well as specific teaching methods, styles, and relationships with clinical experts, students, and colleagues. It should not be seen as a remedial activity, although some faculty may perceive the term as "discounting their level of knowledge or expertise, or as [unfavourable] commentary on the decisions they make about teaching, content, structure, or relationships" (Bevis, 2000, p. 117–118). Rather, faculty development is intended to enhance knowledge and skills. It should evolve naturally as part of the curriculum development process, and be congruent with the institutional philosophy, considerate of faculty needs, and supported by administrators and resources.

Where Does the Responsibility Lie?

The school of nursing dean or director has the responsibility to invest in and support the development of faculty in order to minimize knowledge gaps in curriculum development, teaching, and research. Administrators act as change agents because of their formal leadership positions as deans or directors. They are the primary force in initiating change and assisting faculty in their development (Smolen, 1996).

Identification of specific faculty development needs can be undertaken by the curriculum leader, a committee, or by individual faculty members. Typically, it is a combination of these. It is the responsibility of faculty members to attend faculty development activities, be open to new ideas, participate fully, and commit to employing new knowledge, skills, and perspectives as they develop and implement the curriculum.

Need for Faculty Development

Curriculum development, and ultimately implementation of a new curriculum, is an example of planned change: from a familiar curriculum to one that is initially undefined. Because of faculty members' extensive involvement in curriculum development, implementation plans, and opportunities to introduce aspects of the new curriculum into the current one, the change to a new curriculum might be expected to occur easily and with full faculty support.

Unfortunately, the change is not always smooth. Successful curriculum change is generally dependent on the acquisition of new skills and perspectives by those who will implement the change. Curriculum change requires personal change and this does not happen in a scheduled, orderly fashion, since it evolves according to individual readiness. Faculty development is a means to support change and should take place concurrently with curriculum development. Accordingly, curriculum development mandates faculty development. In turn, faculty development supports curriculum development and change. Figure 4.1 depicts the

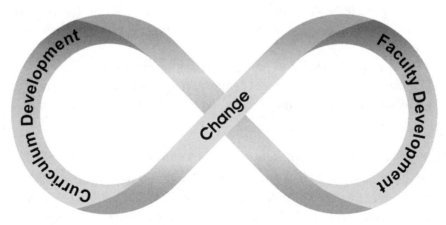

Figure 4.1   Synchronous, Intertwining, and Infinite Nature of Faculty and Curriculum Development

synchronous, infinite, and intertwining nature of faculty development, change, and curriculum development.

Empowerment of Faculty Faculty development has the potential to empower faculty and benefit the school of nursing in ways that extend beyond the tasks of developing and implementing a new curriculum. Rosabeth Moss Kanter (1977) asserts that power (ability to get work done) in organizations is derived from both formal positions and from alliances with superiors, peers, and subordinates. Alliances form the basis of cooperation to get the work done. Formal and informal power give access to opportunity, resources, information, and support. These, in turn, influence employees in positive ways, leading to increased self-efficacy, motivation, organizational commitment, perceived autonomy, perceptions of participative management, and job satisfaction. Burnout is decreased. Employees derive achievement, respect, and cooperation. As well, clients of the organization are satisfied. This theory is relevant for faculty development in schools of nursing.

Within a curriculum development context in schools of nursing, those with formal power are the nursing dean or director, the curriculum leader, and to a lesser extent, those chosen to chair committees. However, many alliances form as work progresses and faculty members derive power from these. More directly, faculty development is a means to provide opportunity, resources, information, and support to faculty, so they can achieve a new curriculum and derive the benefits of it.

Empirical evidence about staff nurse empowerment supports Kanter's (1977) theory (Finegan & Laschinger, 2001; Laschinger, Finegan, & Shamian, 2001; Laschinger, Finegan, Shamian, & Wilk, 2001). The theory has also been tested with nurse educators. Access to opportunity is the most empowering factor for clinical and college nurse educators (Davies, 2002; Sarmiento, Laschinger, & Iwasiw, 2004). Among college educators, empowering environments lead to decreased burnout and increased job satisfaction (Sarmiento, et al.). Unfortunately, college educators view their work environments as only moderately empowering (Erwin, 1999).

Faculty development is needed to support and empower faculty during curriculum development. Planned faculty development demonstrates the school's commitment to faculty and their professional growth, empowers faculty, enhances job satisfaction, and is a means to support change.

Goals for Faculty Development Related to Curriculum Development

"Most faculty development programs are directed toward improving scholarship under the assumption that increased or updated knowledge in faculty's subject fields will lead to improvement in course content" (Dunkley, 1994). However, this is not sufficient when curriculum development is being undertaken. Faculty development goals related to curriculum redesign and development are essentially four-fold. These include enhancing knowledge and skills about curriculum development, and as Bevis (2000) describes, changing views of curriculum, roles and relationships, and teaching approaches. All the aforementioned goals are equally important and are achieved synergistically.

Enhancing Knowledge and Skills About Curriculum Development   Knowledge about the curriculum development process varies among faculty members and other stakeholders. Some will know a great deal; others will be familiar with details of course planning, but not with the larger process. Likely, many will have learning needs related to the developing curriculum. To make certain that the curriculum development process is smooth, faculty development focused specifically on developing a curriculum is necessary. Knowledge of the total process will lead to an appreciation of the time required for curriculum development, work accomplished by task groups, and importance of shared understandings and consensus. Moreover, detailed information about each aspect of curriculum development will allow task groups to develop their critical paths and ensure work is completed in the manner required.

Changing View of Curriculum   Another goal for faculty development is acceptance of a different perception of curriculum and learning. In the past, learning was generally accepted as simply a change in behavior, dependent on content. Currently, learning is seen as evolving from transactions and interactions between and among students and teachers, which culminate from the curriculum. This latter connotation is less reliant on content, more oriented to the process of nursing, and is a more egalitarian view of curriculum, with "teaching goals…[that] lead to creative and critical thinking, strategizing, and methods of inquiry consistent with learner maturity" (Bevis, 2000, p. 123). Although many nurse educators have enthusiastically endorsed this perspective over the last two decades, faculty could consider other approaches. For example, curricula could be conceived phenomenologically, ethically, narratively, contextually, or clinically. Whichever approach to curriculum is adopted, it is important to facilitate faculty members' understanding about the selected view and provide faculty development opportunities such as workshops, conferences, and mentoring to assist them in designing curricula reflecting the new view.

Changing Roles and Relationships   A change in faculty roles could be a consequence of a new or revised curriculum, and this would mean altered relationships with students, colleagues, administrators, and clients. The role change might involve a shift in power, equity, and authority, depending on the philosophical approaches and goals of the curriculum. Faculty facing new and/or revised roles resulting from curriculum change can be helped through faculty development activities which incorporate sensitivity training, sharing, nurturing, and consciousness raising (Wheeler, & Chinn, 1989).

Changing Teaching Approaches   A realistic goal of faculty development is to encourage nurse educators to become more aware of how they teach, and how they might teach more effectively. To help them do so, activities (e.g., role playing, case studies, practice teaching and critiques, videos or films with discussion), as well as psychological support and encouragement could be employed. The purpose is to assist *novice* faculty to acquire teaching skills, and *experienced* faculty to revitalize their current teaching practices and courses (Davis, 1993) to be congruent with the new curriculum. Faculty development activities to support changed teaching approaches should be considered in light of curriculum philosophical approaches and goals.

Faculty Development Activities for Curriculum Development

Faculty engaging in curriculum development may require additional knowledge and skills about the process they are undertaking. This learning can be facilitated through planned faculty development activities such as workshops, mentoring, group discussions, and attendance at conferences. See Table 4.1 for examples of formal and informal strategies for faculty development that could be relevant for faculty development related to curriculum development.

Faculty development programs should be ongoing, but quite naturally assume more importance when a new curriculum is envisioned. Whether faculty development activities are formal or informal, the focus should be on the curriculum development process itself. It be-

TABLE 4.1 STRATEGIES FOR FORMAL AND INFORMAL FACULTY DEVELOPMENT

Strategies	
Formal	**Informal**
• Center for faculty development	• One-on-one
• Inservice workshops	• Dialogue and feedback
• Lectures and formal conferences by experts and/or experienced colleagues	• Meetings with department heads
	• Handbooks
• Post-graduate courses	• Mentorship
• Forums	• Preceptorship
• Seminars	• Buddy system
• Learning studies laboratory	• Learning circles
• Faculty meetings	• Luncheon meetings
• Practice teaching	• Support groups
• Integrative partnerships	• Readings
• Group meetings	• Audiovisual and computer programs
• Tours, visits	• Modeling
• Retreats	• Shadowing
	• Tutoring

gins with organizing for curriculum change, and includes collecting and interpreting contextual data, establishing curriculum directions, goals, and philosophical approaches, designing curriculum and courses, and evaluating curriculum. Notably, inherent in the design and implementation of a faculty development program is a faculty vision of themselves ". . . as the planners and power persons with the opportunity to plan, practice, and perfect new teaching roles . . . and new alliances with students and practice persons" (Bevis & Murray, 1990, p. 131).

Curriculum developers should meet initially in faculty development sessions to gain an overview of the curriculum development process. It is incumbent upon all stakeholders to reach shared understandings about nursing education, nursing and health care, teaching-learning processes and student-teacher-practitioner relationships. Faculty discussions of this nature serve the added purpose of moving the curriculum development process forward.

Because faculty development is ongoing, a schedule must be agreed upon. Each session's topic, format, time, location, and leader need to be decided early. However, schedules and topics should not be so fixed that changes cannot be instituted to meet participant obligations, newly identified or urgent needs, and other contingencies. Nonetheless, what must be kept in mind is that in order to design and develop a curriculum that will be acceptable to all stakeholders and relevant at the time of curriculum implementation and beyond, faculty development is necessary. Faculty must come together, learn and grow together, accept that change is inevitable, and take ownership and pride in the future. Individuals who participate in faculty development feel:

- valued in an organization that invests in curriculum development participants
- competent because of attainment of new abilities and progress toward goal achievement
- secure in group learning and interaction
- empowered by the institution's interest in their professional development and provision of opportunities, resources, information, and support
- and connected to colleagues through shared learning, acceptance, appreciation, and respect

Faculty Development for Curriculum Change

Faculty may experience feelings ranging from anticipation to resistance as the existing curriculum ends and the transition to the new curriculum takes place (Kupperschmidt & Burns, 1997). Faculty development is intended to support faculty members' personal and professional growth when a new curriculum is envisioned, curriculum work begins, and curriculum change occurs. Therefore, consideration of how faculty might undergo change is a significant element of faculty development. Activities to support faculty during a curriculum change merit attention. Strategies to respond to resisters in order to enhance their participation in faculty development and acceptance of the new curriculum direction are also important. The following brief section on change theories is foundational to understanding how to support faculty and respond to resistance to curriculum change.

Change Theories

Lewin's Force-Field Analysis Kurt Lewin describes change as a social-psychological process with three phases: unfreezing, moving, and refreezing. In the *unfreezing phase*, a problem or desired change is identified, and a force field analysis is conducted to determine the driving and restraining forces. Together, the leader and the target group examine the issue, and develop strategies and actions to minimize the forces limiting change and maximize the forces driving the change. In the *moving phase*, actions are carried out as the system moves toward the desired state. Finally, in the *refreezing phase*, the change is stabilized in both individuals and the system (Lewin, as cited in Skelton-Green, 1999; Sullivan & Decker, 2001).

Rogers and Shoemaker's Diffusion of Change Rogers and Shoemaker (as cited in Skelton-Green, 1999) propose a three-phase model of change: *invention* of the change; *diffusion* or *communication* of information about the change; and *consequence*, which can be acceptance or rejection of the change. This model is premised on the assumption that people are rational and therefore, knowledge will lead logically to acceptance of a proposed change. Accordingly, communication about all aspects of the change and the intended outcomes are fundamental to success. People involved in the change are characterized below, according to their readiness for change.

- Innovators seek change
- Early adapters facilitate change
- Early majority members provide a support system for change
- Late majority members exert peer pressure to support the change
- Laggards strive to maintain the status quo
- Rejecters actively oppose the change

Transtheoretical Model of Behavior Change This model addresses behavior change of an individual as the desired outcome, and incorporates changes in attitudes, intentions, and behavior. Behavioral change is conceptualized as a spiral and this pattern represents the reality that people do not change in a straightforward, linear manner. Rather, at certain times, individuals can revert to former stages, and then proceed again toward the desired change. The stages represent a continuum of motivational readiness. Relapse to previous stages is considered a natural part of the change cycle. The stages are:

- precontemplation: person sees no need to change
- contemplation: person thinks about the benefits and losses of change and admits to desiring change, but there is no intent to act
- preparation: person plans to make a specific change soon, and may make small attempts at change
- action: person makes an overt commitment to change and practices the new behavior over time
- maintenance: person is able to avoid relapses to former stages for six months or more, although the temptation to relapse can persist for several years (Prochaska, DiClemente, & Norcross, 1992; Prochaska, Redding, Harlow, Rossi, & Velicer, 1994)

Participation in faculty and curriculum development can be conceptualized as encompassing a change in faculty attitude toward the current curriculum, an intention to create a new curriculum, and a change in behavior to include curriculum development activities. Curriculum implementation, then, requires a change in attitude toward students, other faculty, and roles; an intention to behave and interact in new ways; and a change in teaching behavior, approach to content, and interactions. Faculty development activities provide the knowledge, skills, and environment that support individual and collective change. Participation in faculty development represents action to change attitudes and behavior.

Supporting Faculty During Curriculum Change

Development of a new curriculum, while faculty are concurrently fulfilling teaching and research responsibilities, requires their dedication to a new vision, and tangible organizational support. Faculty development is one form of substantive support. In Table 4.2, the Model of Behavior Change (Prochaska et al., 1992; Prochaska et al., 1994) is applied to faculty and curriculum change, with activities proposed to match the stages of the model. Incorporated into the strategies, and indeed within the curriculum development process itself, are factors that are inherently empowering: publicity about activities; strong relationship between activities and a central issue in the organization; high interpersonal contact; and participation in programs, meetings, and problem-solving groups (Kanter, 1997). The school must invest in the faculty, and the faculty members, in turn, will invest themselves in the school and its future.

Responding to Resistance to Change

Chapter 2 presented some ideas about responding to initial objections to curriculum change through an appeal to values and logic. Even though a school of nursing proceeds with

TABLE 4.2   APPLICATION OF TRANSTHEORETICAL MODEL OF BEHAVIOR CHANGE TO FACULTY AND CURRICULUM CHANGE

Stage of Change	Process of Change for Faculty	Activities to Support Faculty and Curriculum Change
Precontemplation: no intention to change	Consciousness-raising (increasing level of awareness and more accurate information-processing)	• Present data about need for curriculum change • Engage faculty in discussion about the possibility of curriculum change
	Dramatic relief (experiencing and expressing feelings)	• Stimulate faculty discussion about frustrations and disappointments experienced within the current curriculum
	Environmental re-evaluation (affective and cognitive re-experiencing of one's environment and problems)	• Initiate faculty discussion to identify features of the current curriculum they dislike
Contemplation: seriously considering a curriculum change within a specified time	Consciousness-raising	• Continue discussion about the need for curriculum change • Engage faculty in consideration of the benefits of curriculum change
	Dramatic relief	• Use guided imagery for faculty to imagine how they will feel when an up-to-date, well-received curriculum is in place
	Environmental re-evaluation	• Share ideas about the effects of avoiding curriculum change on students, graduates, school of nursing, and educational institution

Preparation: a commitment has been made to change the curriculum

Self-re-evaluation (affective and cognitive re-experiencing of one's self and problems)

- Initiate deliberations among faculty and dean or director about the possibility of removing barriers to faculty involvement in curriculum development
- Review school and university mission and goals and how strongly the current curriculum supports mission and goals
- Plan discussion about faculty values related to education, nursing practice, profession
- Identify initial faculty development needs

Environmental re-evaluation*

- Minimize barriers and maximize resources for faculty and curriculum development
- Obtain agreement from the Total Faculty Group to proceed with curriculum development
- Declare administrator support publicly
- Announce curriculum development plans to stakeholders
- Appoint curriculum leader

Self-liberation (belief in one's ability to change and commitment to act on that belief)

- Form Steering and Advisory Committees
- Initiate faculty development activities
- Establish committees and obtain agreement from members to achieve goals

continues

TABLE 4.2   CONTINUED

Stage of Change	Process of Change for Faculty	Activities to Support Faculty and Curriculum Change
Action: active engagement in: • curriculum development • faculty development • testing of new faculty behaviors in the current curriculum	Reinforcement management (reinforcing more positive behaviors and punishing negative ones)	• Develop critical path • Institute mentorship • Provide positive feedback to individuals and committees • Provide rewards for faculty and curriculum development activities (e.g., public acknowledgment and praise, credit toward promotion and tenure) • Celebrate achievement of major milestones of critical path • Continue formal and informal faculty development and support (e.g., teaching circles, lunch discussions, on-line discussion groups, peer feedback) • Use new terminology • Introduce aspects of new curriculum into old curriculum
	Self-liberation*	• Mentor novices • Continue faculty development activities focused on faculty self-identified needs • Identify and acknowledge experts in school of nursing • Conduct a funeral for the old curriculum

Maintenance: sustained behavior	Counter-conditioning (substituting more positive behaviors and experiences for problem ones)	• Continue faculty development based on experiences in testing new behaviors and implementing new curriculum
		• Structure formal evaluation of faculty and courses to be congruent with new curriculum

		• Disseminate information about the new curriculum to:
		  • academic and professional communities
		  • prospective students

	Stimulus control (restructuring environment or experiences so that problem stimuli are less likely to occur)	• Launch new curriculum with a public celebration
		• Ask for counter-examples of effective strategies if objections arise or reversion to former curriculum occurs
		• Encourage peer groups to support new faculty behaviors and curriculum implementation
	Helping relationships (relationships involving openness, caring, trust, genuineness, and empathy)	• Continue peer faculty development and support activities through group activities and mentorship
		• Schedule formal faculty development for aspects of curriculum implementation that are problematic. Focus on shared problem-solving

continues

TABLE 4.2   CONTINUED

Stage of Change	Process of Change for Faculty	Activities to Support Faculty and Curriculum Change
	Self-re-evaluation*	• Share stories abut "how far we've come" and identify new values, beliefs, and aspirations • Use teaching portfolios for faculty evaluation (self, peer, and administrator)

*processes not identified in these stages in original Transtheoretical Model
[Some data from: Prochaska, J.O., DiClemente, C.C., & Norcross, J.C. (1992). In search of how people change: Applications to addictive behaviors. *American Psychologist, 47,* 1102–1114; and Prochaska, J.O., Redding, C.A., Harlow, L.L., Rossi, J.S., & Velicer, W.F. (1994). The transtheoretical model of change and HIV prevention: A review. *Health Education Quarterly, 21,* 471–486.]

curriculum development, there may be some members who do not agree with the need for change or faculty development. Although a minority group, resisters have the potential to undermine the momentum of the majority. This cannot be allowed. Every effort should be extended to help the resisters feel that their contributions are needed and valued, and to counteract the negativity that they might project. There is a diplomatic balance to be achieved between sensitivity to individual readiness for change and the school's need to progress with faculty and curriculum development.

Forms and Causes of Resistance *Active resistance* to curriculum change and faculty development is easy to identify. Examples of active resistance include:

- open criticism of curriculum change and faculty development
- refusal to acknowledge shortcomings of the present curriculum or need for faculty development
- predictions of dire consequences of curriculum change
- direct refusal to participate in faculty and curriculum development

Passive resistance is subtler. Although resisting participation in faculty or curriculum development, the passive resister lacks the courage to openly state opposition. Behavior typical of passive resistance can be:

- lateness for, or absence from, meetings
- failure to meet commitments to complete work
- minimal participation in activities attended
- diverting attention from the main purpose of meetings to trivial, peripheral, or historical matters

Passive-aggressive resistance is sabotage. The resister publicly supports faculty development and curriculum change, and is involved in these activities. Yet, this endorsement is coupled with behind-the-scenes attempts to undermine faculty development plans, the proposed curriculum, and/or those participating in faculty and curriculum development.

Responding to Resistance The source of resistance must be determined in order to respond effectively. This can be difficult if the source is related to self-concept or motivation, even when trusting relationships exist among faculty. Ignoring the resistance is to condone it (Chambers, 1998). The administrator should:

- invite the resister to a private meeting, so that the resistance can be addressed directly
- employ exemplary listening skills so the resister feels heard
- clearly state expectations about:
  - participating in faculty development

- participating in curriculum development
- teaching according to new tenets
- accepting consequences of not meeting expectations

Responding to Publicly Voiced Criticism Particularly troubling are reports of a faculty member's public criticism of faculty development and curriculum change. Responses should convey respect for the resister and confidence in faculty development and the future curriculum. Appropriate comments might be:

- "The new curriculum will maintain our tradition of excellence. One way we are ensuring this is through our faculty development."
- "We are receiving solid support for the proposed curriculum from practitioners and nursing leaders, and are working hard to ensure that we will be ready to implement our new approaches."

Public criticism of the developing curriculum is not acceptable and should be directly addressed with the faculty member. The goal is to obtain the resister's agreement to refrain from further public criticism. The school leader needs to be precise, objective, and unemotional in describing the reports and their effects on the members and image of the school. The dean or director should convey the following messages:

- The curriculum is changing and the opportunity to influence the curriculum is now
- There could be consequences of not participating (e.g., isolation from colleagues, unsatisfactory performance appraisal)
- Future teaching performance will be evaluated in accordance with the intent of the new curriculum

In this way, the resister can have no doubts about present and future expectations. The discussion can be concluded with a statement about the resister's strengths and an invitation to contribute these strengths to faculty and curriculum development. Possible responses to reasons for resistance to faculty development and curriculum change, are presented in Table 4.3.

An Alternate Perspective To lessen the stress often experienced when resistance is prolonged or unrelenting, it may be helpful to reframe the situation to make the discord or dissent seem less personal. Viewing resistance as a conflict of values, beliefs, rights, and obligations could lead to changed understandings and reactions by all involved. Table 4.4 presents examples of possible areas of conflict and possible perspectives of resisters and the faculty majority. A different perspective and emotional distance may make the situation more tolerable, and lessen the tendency to view the resister as a villain. Explicit use of conflict resolution strategies may be in order.

TABLE 4.3   POSSIBLE RESPONSES TO REASONS FOR RESISTANCE TO FACULTY DEVELOPMENT AND CURRICULUM CHANGE

Reasons for Resistance to Faculty Development and Curriculum Change	Possible Responses of Administrator, Curriculum Leader, and/or Faculty Majority
Belief in value of current curriculum and way of being	• Explore which aspects of curriculum and role are valued and why. • Suggest that involvement in faculty and curriculum development is the best way to ensure continuation of what is valued. • Make evident how aspects of current curriculum might be taken into account in the developing curriculum.
Skepticism about quality of envisioned curriculum	• Explore concerns. • Be open to possibility that resister is correct. • Acknowledge that the resister's input has assisted in the examination of the issue, along with others' views.
Interpretation of change as personal criticism	• Validate the progressive nature of current curriculum at the time it was developed. • Explain in detail the need for a changed curriculum. • Emphasize what will be gained by changed curricular and faculty approaches. • Listen actively to resister's issues (e.g., losses, fears), and if possible, attempt to lessen the frequency of verbalization of concerns. • Emphasize that the resister's strengths are needed for faculty and curriculum development activities. • Validate the resister's past contributions and express confidence in ability to be successful.

continues

TABLE 4.3   CONTINUED

Reasons for Resistance to Faculty Development and Curriculum Change	Possible Responses of Administrator, Curriculum Leader, and/or Faculty Majority
Belief in own curriculum development expertise; hence no need for faculty development	• Acknowledge experience and knowledge that resister has accumulated. • Propose that resister share expertise by leading some faculty development sessions. Assign this as part of workload, if possible. • State consequences of non-participation.
Fear of reduced status or not fitting into new curriculum	• Emphasize that all faculty are uncertain about their place in the changed curriculum, particularly in the early stages when the new curriculum is undefined. • Encourage participation in faculty and curriculum development as a means of ensuring that a place can be identified and developed in the future curriculum. • Stress that faculty development activities will prepare all faculty for the envisioned curriculum.
Fear that inadequate skills and knowledge will be revealed	• Relate anecdotes from school or personal history when faculty felt that they could not succeed in changed circumstances, yet did achieve. • Propose the idea that many faculty may wonder if they "have what it takes" to function in the changed curriculum. • Assure that school director attends faculty development activities to underscore that everyone has learning needs and to give importance to attendance.
Lack of confidence in colleagues' ability to develop acceptable curriculum	• Agree that not all faculty are equally experienced in nursing education generally, and in curriculum development particularly.

- Underscore that the curriculum development process is inherently a form of faculty development, and therefore colleagues will enhance skills as the project unfolds.
- Emphasize that formal and informal faculty development will occur concurrently with curriculum development, thereby expanding colleagues' skills and knowledge.
- Indicate that curriculum development is an opportunity for the resister to share particular expertise in nursing education, thereby becoming a model for less-experienced faculty.

Lack of confidence in own ability to contribute meaningfully

- Emphasize that all faculty are uncertain about undertaking curriculum development.
- Remind resister that ongoing faculty development is intended to ensure that all faculty will have access to pertinent perspectives and be able to contribute to curriculum work.
- Relate strengths that resister can bring to curriculum development.

Lack of interest or disinclination to expend effort required for faculty development, curriculum change and implementation

- Explore reasons and remove barriers if possible.
- Remind resister that faculty and curriculum development are shared responsibilities of all faculty.
- Discuss how resister expects to be effective in changed curriculum if not involved in its creation and in faculty development.
- Employ all strategies to help resister feel that contributions are needed and valued.
- Consider an alternate assignment in the school of nursing, as a last resort or if retirement is imminent.

continues

TABLE 4.3   CONTINUED

Reasons for Resistance to Faculty Development and Curriculum Change	Possible Responses of Administrator, Curriculum Leader, and/or Faculty Majority
Concern that faculty and curriculum development will interfere with research and publication and/or progress towards tenure	• Acknowledge that faculty and curriculum development require intensive effort. • Discuss research and publication potential of curriculum development and implementation. • Describe how curriculum development can contribute to promotion and tenure. • Consider the feasibility of some faculty "opting out" of curriculum development for short periods at critical points of research activity or career progress.
Heavy workload	• Examine how workload could be altered to include participation in faculty and curriculum development activities.
Misoneism (fear of newness, innovation, or change)	• Provide as much support as possible to enhance motivation for change. • Accept that no one can cause another to change.
Unrevealed personal reasons	• Accept that it is not possible to respond constructively to what is unknown.

TABLE 4.4   POSSIBLE PERSPECTIVES ON CONFLICT AREAS ABOUT NEED FOR FACULTY AND CURRICULUM DEVELOPMENT

Possible Conflict Areas	Possible Perspective on Conflict Areas	
	Resister	Faculty Majority
Values	• Stability • Experience • Personal values	• Change • Personal growth • Shared values
Beliefs	• Quality education = current curriculum, teaching, and evaluation methods • Personal value as a teacher and nurse is expressed in current curriculum • Faculty development and curriculum change are a repudiation of current practices	• Quality education = changed curriculum, teaching, and evaluation methods • Future curriculum will enhance growth as teachers and nurses • Faculty development and curriculum change will expand and enhance knowledge and skills
Interpretation of the right of academic freedom	• Criticism • Individual decision-making about curriculum	• Critique • Collegial decision-making and adherence to curriculum decisions made by Total Faculty Group
Obligations	• Maintenance of present programs • Adherence to current (correct) way of doing things • Preparation of graduates for existing nursing practice	• Planning and implementation of a relevant and progressive program • Openness to new ideas • Preparation of graduates for future nursing practice

Faculty are responsible for their own reactions and behaviors. Some may choose to reject faculty and curriculum development and curricular changes, content to be miserable and out of step with colleagues, despite efforts to support them through change. When faced with such individuals, it is paramount to remember that you cannot change others. However, it is possible and may be necessary to change your reaction so that you are not consumed with anxiety, anger, and the endless creation of appeasement tactics. Focus on the task at hand: prepare for a new curriculum with motivated, growth-seeking colleagues.

Chapter Summary

Faculty development is an essential component of curriculum development. Identifying learning needs and planning activities that will enhance knowledge and skills as stakeholders move through the curriculum development process will maximize opportunities for a successful change. A wide spectrum of faculty development activities should be considered and the most suitable selected. However, it is realistic to acknowledge that not all faculty may welcome empowerment and change; some might be very comfortable with maintaining the status quo. Helping faculty achieve a common understanding that roles and relationships, or teaching approaches, could change because of the new or revised curriculum, and encouraging them to take an active part in development activities can be challenging, but ultimately rewarding. Nevertheless, proceeding with a planned faculty development program as it relates to curriculum development and change is important and should not be delayed.

Synthesis Activities

Two cases are presented to illustrate the main ideas of the chapter. The first is critiqued and the second is followed by questions to help with analysis. Questions at the end of this section of the chapter are intended to assist with faculty development related to curriculum development.

Copernicus University School of Nursing

Copernicus University, a mid-size university with a long history, houses several world-renowned programs. Of these, astronomy and nursing are held in high esteem for their progressive ideas. Over the last few months, and after much deliberation, faculty came to the realization that a curriculum revision would be in order. They agreed that the curriculum, as currently designed, was too structured and no longer reflected their evolving beliefs about teaching, learning, and the nursing profession.

The faculty, under the leadership of Dr. Korsan, have had many discussions about how the current philosophical basis of the curriculum does not match their desire for a more phenomenological approach to teaching nursing and providing patient care. They believe that the essence of lived experiences of learners and clients, along with faculty views, should shape the curriculum. All faculty were supportive of this direction and many ideas were shared about how to proceed. Two task forces were struck. The responsibility of the first was to thoroughly research the concept of phenomenology and what implications this philosophical approach would have on revising the existing curriculum. The second was to search for and examine existing curricula grounded in phenomenology, as well as other approaches that incorporate lived experiences. These committees were to report back to the Total Faculty Group in two months.

The task forces did their research on phenomenology, examined other programs that used this and other approaches, and held small focus groups with faculty in each year of the program. Findings were shared and many issues raised at a faculty meeting. The predominant concern was whether it was premature to select the philosophical approach without having a thorough understanding of what other options might be possible. After considerable deliberation, faculty concurred that although a change was desirable, they would benefit from some planned faculty development sessions about several philosophical approaches, and an examination of what engaging in curriculum revision of this nature would mean to them.

The faculty decided that a retreat would be the best way to proceed. Dr. Korsan agreed to hire an expert for a one-day, off-campus retreat for faculty and other stakeholders. Another faculty member thought it wise to strike a faculty development committee to plan future learning opportunities in an organized and strategic fashion. There was overall agreement for this idea and the dean asked faculty to think about whether they would like to serve on this committee.

Critique Copernicus University School of Nursing has a cohesive faculty committed to changing the undergraduate curriculum. Motivation for change came from the total faculty, who are willing to participate in task forces and focus groups, and complete literature searches. Faculty involvement is valued. Their concerns about a new direction as well as suggestions about how to proceed are respected. It is likely that the collective strength of faculty will support them through their desired change and facilitate feelings of ownership of the proposed changes as the process unfolds.

The collective decision to proceed carefully by learning more about several philosophical approaches for nursing curricula is sensible. Faculty members believe that a change is desirable. They feel a need to focus more on lived experiences of clients, learners, and themselves; however, they do not fully understand what this change may imply or how to go about introducing it. Consideration will have to be given to faculty's knowledge about the process of curriculum redesign. Other issues, such as how the curriculum should be developed to assure congruence with the curriculum goals, have not yet been identified. Whether curriculum revision is a process with which they are familiar or one with which they have had little experience, this assessment is required. It is likely that as faculty progress with curriculum development, many learning needs will arise related to roles and relationships, curriculum implementation, teaching, and evaluation. It will be important to assess their understanding about how to implement the proposed changes in the curriculum and what implications these could have for all stakeholders.

Dr. Korsan is demonstrating commitment to the process by supporting a formal faculty development opportunity facilitated by an expert, so faculty can gain a more complete understanding of philosophical approaches as these apply to nursing curricula. This is a good start. As well, Copernicus University School of Nursing has wisely decided to form a faculty development committee. Striking this committee will maintain momentum and continue to move the process forward. The group will be able to use the data collected to plan further learning opportunities. It will be prudent for the committee to ascertain faculty needs and preferred strategies, as well as the resources available to implement the plans they propose. The school's approach to adopting a new philosophical direction and the plan to proceed is being carefully executed.

Rosemount University School of Nursing

Rosemount University School of Nursing has offered baccalaureate and masters programs in nursing for 40 years. Most faculty have kept abreast of changing curriculum paradigms and teaching methods in order to deliver the "best" nursing program to qualified students. Faculty development through attendance at occasional in-house meetings or attendance at local, national, or international conferences has been considered important to most of the faculty. However, an ongoing faculty development program was not implemented due to resistance from a few "senior" faculty members.

Recently, Dr. Angela Fabatini, director of the school, attended a national meeting of baccalaureate nursing program deans and directors. One recommendation, among many others developed by the group, was that faculty development include activities intended to facilitate participation in curriculum development.

On returning from the conference, Dr. Fabatini called a faculty meeting. A review of current faculty development activities was undertaken. The results revealed a fragmented approach to faculty development, sporadic faculty attendance, and very little attention to the specifics of the curriculum process. Inexperienced faculty members expressed the need for an ongoing faculty development program to assist them in revising the present baccalaureate-nursing program. Two "senior" experienced faculty members voiced their resistance to this activity, claiming that the past practice of ad hoc meetings was satisfactory and that there was no need for change, since the program is accredited.

Questions for Consideration and Analysis of Rosemount University Case

1. What are the strengths and limitations in the present faculty development system?
2. What strategies might be instituted to encourage participation in faculty development?
3. When agreement is reached to undertake faculty development for curriculum change, what would be the goals of this activity? What development activities could be instituted?

4. What responses might be appropriate for those faculty members resisting change?

5. Which change theory would be useful, and how could it be implemented?

Curriculum Development Activities for Consideration in Your Setting

To plan for faculty development related to curriculum development in your setting, consider the questions below:

1. Who could best champion the faculty development process in your institution?

2. What might be the anticipated and unanticipated benefits and challenges associated with initiating faculty development activities in your setting?

3. Which faculty development activities do faculty currently accept or reject?

4. How can faculty be supported to view curriculum development as an engaging and empowering process?

5. Consider the elements of the Transtheoretical Model of Behavior Change. According to these elements, which activities do you believe would be most constructive in helping faculty move smoothly through the transition from the current to the envisioned curriculum?

6. What resources (human, physical, material, fiscal) can the school access to support faculty development initiatives during curriculum development?

7. What are the key elements of a faculty development program to support faculty development and curriculum change in your school?

8. Design a faculty development program for your school of nursing.

References

Bevis, E.O. (2000). Clusters of influence for practical decision making about curriculum. In E.O. Bevis, & J. Watson (Eds.), *Toward a caring curriculum: A new pedagogy for nursing.* (pp. 107–152). Boston: Jones and Bartlett Publishers.

Bevis, E.O., & Murray, J.P. (1990). The essence of curriculum revolution: Emancipatory teaching. *Journal of Nursing Education, 29,* 326–331.

Chambers, H.E. (1998). *The Bad Attitude Survival Guide.* Reading, Massachusetts: Addison-Wesley.

Davies, M.A. (2002). *Perceived workplace empowerment, job tension, and job satisfaction of clinical educators in hospital settings: Testing Kanter's theory.* University of Western Ontario, London, Ontario, Canada, Unpublished master's thesis.

Davis, B. (1993). *Tools for teaching.* San Francisco: Jossey-Bass Publishers.

Dunkley, N.A. (1994). How do you want to improve yourself? Nursing administration and faculty attitudes toward types of faculty development. *Journal of Continuing Education in Nursing, 25,* 277–281.

Erwin, E.M. (1999). *The relationships between perceptions of workplace empowerment of college nurse educators and an organizational climate for caring in the workplace.* University of Western Ontario, London, Ontario, Canada, Unpublished master's thesis.

Finegan, J.E., & Laschinger, H.K.S. (2001). The antecedents and consequences of empowerment. *Journal of Nursing Administration, 31,* 489–497.

Halliburton, D., Marincovich, M., & Svinicki, M. (1988). Strengthening professional development. *Journal of Higher Education, 59*(3), 291–304.

Kanter, R.M. (1977). *Men and women of the corporation.* New York: Basic Books.

Kupperschmidt, B.R., & Burns, P. (1997). Curriculum revision isn't just change: it's transition! *Journal of Professional Nursing, 13,* 90–98.

Laschinger, H.K.S., Finegan, J., & Shamian, J. (2001). The impact of workplace empowerment, organizational trust on staff nurses' work satisfaction and organizational commitment. *Health Care Management Review, 26*(3), 7–23.

Laschinger, H.K.S., Finegan, J., Shamian, J., & Wilk, P. (2001). Impact of structural and psychological empowerment on job strain in work settings: Expanding Kanter's Theory. *Journal of Nursing Administration, 31,* 260–272.

Prochaska, J.O., DiClemente, C.C., & Norcross, J.C. (1992). In search of how people change: Applications to addictive behaviors. *American Psychologist, 47,* 1102–1114.

Prochaska, J.O., Redding, C.A., Harlow, L.L., Rossi, J.S., & Velicer, W.F. (1994). The transtheoretical model of change and HIV prevention: A review. *Health Education Quarterly, 21,* 471–486.

Rush, K., Ouellet, L., & Wasson, D. (1991). Faculty development: The essence of curriculum development. *Nurse Education Today, 11,* 121–126.

Sarmiento, T., Laschinger, H.K.S., & Iwasiw, C. (2004). College educators' workplace empowerment, burnout, and job satisfaction: Testing Kanter's theory. *Journal of Advanced Nursing, 24,* 134–143.

Skelton-Green, J. (1999). Managing change. In J.M. Hibberd & D.L. Smith, *Nursing Management in Canada.* (2nd ed.) (pp. 455–470). Toronto: W. B. Saunders Canada.

Smolen, D. (1996). Constraints that nursing program administrators encounter in promoting faculty change and development. *Journal of Professional Nursing, 12*(2), 91–98.

Sullivan, E.J., & Decker, P.J. (2001). *Effective Leadership and Management in Nursing, 5th ed.* Prentice-Hall: Upper Saddle River, New Jersey.

Wheeler, C.E., & Chinn, P.L. (1989). *Peace and power, a handbook of feminist process.* New York: National League for Nursing.

CHAPTER 5

Gathering Data About Contextual Factors for Curriculum Development

Chapter Overview

Contextual factors, both within and beyond the school of nursing, must be investigated if the new curriculum is to be progressive, relevant, and congruent with institutional goals and societal needs. Although the contextual factors can be viewed in many ways, the typology of contextual factors in this chapter presents a reasonable way to conceptualize them. These contextual factors have a major influence on curriculum. Following a discussion about the influence of the factors on the curriculum, important internal and external contextual factors are described. Then, practical approaches to gathering data are outlined, including considerations to help determine essential data, the data sources to pursue, and methods to obtain the data. Additionally, faculty development pertinent to gathering data about contextual factors is described. A case study and critique exemplify the important points of the chapter and a second case is presented for analysis. Finally, questions are included to determine readiness to undertake data gathering activities.

Chapter Goals

- Appreciate how contextual factors influence curriculum development
- Identify internal and external contextual factors that influence curriculum directions

- Determine essential data to gather about the contextual factors
- Explore data gathering methods and data sources relevant to curriculum development
- Consider faculty development activities related to gathering data about contextual factors

Influence of Contextual Factors on Curriculum Development

Contextual factors are those forces, situations, and circumstances that exist both within and outside the school of nursing and have the potential to influence the school and its programs. The contextual factors are inter-related, complex, and ever-changing. The forces, situations, and circumstances can be as intangible as the ethos of the community's main health care agency and as concrete as the school's budget.

For the purposes of curriculum development, *internal contextual factors* are those forces, situations, and circumstances that originate within the school and educational institution, that is, within the internal environment of the educational institution. *External contextual factors* are those forces, situations, and circumstances that originate outside the educational institution in the community, region, country, and world.

Because the contextual factors (e.g., socio-politico-economics) can be large, nebulous, and/or seamless, curriculum developers must define precisely which data are needed about the factors. The *data* foundational to curriculum development are the specific facts and information about the contextual factors deemed most likely to shape the curriculum. These data might be as specific as graduates' scores on licensure examinations or as imprecise as employers' impressions about graduates' ability to assume new roles. Clearly, the more definitive the data, the stronger the foundation for identifying curriculum directions.

Although differentiated for the purpose of descriptive clarity, in reality some internal and external contextual factors blend, intermingle, and overlap. As well, some factors exist in both internal and external environments. For example, *culture* can be viewed as an internal contextual factor when reviewed in relation to the school of nursing, and as an external contextual factor when described in relation to the community. An examination of the contextual factors within and across the internal and external environments provides curriculum developers with current information from which they can infer future trends about:

- characteristics of learners
- learning expectations and environments
- professional practice expectations and environments
- clients of nursing care

- major health problems and risks
- societal characteristics and needs

Organized, comprehensive, and accurate information about contextual factors is essential to develop a curriculum that:

- can be implemented within the realities of the school and community, now and for the next decade
- incorporates future-oriented thinking about nursing education
- is consistent with the priorities and directions of the educational institution
- is designed to attract and retain faculty and students
- will be responsive to trends in the nursing profession, the community, health care, and society

Internal Contextual Factors

The internal contextual factors are those forces, situations, and circumstances that originate within the school of nursing and educational institution. These include the history, philosophy, culture, financial resources, programs, and infrastructure of the school and institution. When embarking on curriculum development, faculty should be acutely aware of the factors that influence curriculum.

History

Examining the institution's history will reveal past values, successes, and challenges, as well as the school's processes for curriculum development. Much can be learned about how past challenges have been met and successes achieved. This information may still be pertinent for decisions about the curriculum. For example, if the educational institution is one that has built an international reputation, curriculum developers might examine the way this was done, and ask how the nursing curriculum could contribute to or capitalize on this renown. Answers to the following questions will provide some insight into the history of the school of nursing and the institution.

- When were the educational institution and the school of nursing started, and why?
- Have the institution's and school's purposes changed over time? If so, why?
- How does the history influence current programs and operations?
- What programs are offered? How have these evolved? Over what time frame?

- Were programs developed for a niche market?
- What are the unique features that have developed within the institution, the school, and the programs?

When preparing a new curriculum, faculty are creating the school's history. The processes should be recorded for future curriculum developers.

Philosophy, Mission, and Goals

Institutions of higher education have clearly articulated guiding principles, or beliefs and values, about the services offered, the community served, and the fundamental activities that take place within them. Statements about education, learning, knowledge development, scholarship, and so forth form the philosophy. Before initiating curriculum development, faculty require a solid understanding of the educational institution's philosophy and fundamental guiding principles. The nursing curriculum must be congruent with these.

In addition to understanding the institution's philosophy, it is important to identify the guiding principles that operate within the school of nursing. Examining the strength of adherence to the publicly espoused school philosophy will allow for inferences about how easily faculty will accept and implement another one.

Every organization has a mission and a philosophical direction. The mission is a succinct statement that informs those within and outside the organization of its ultimate raison d'être, goals, and direction. The educational institution's mission shapes the nature, scope, and boundaries of the school's direction, goals, and curricula.

The mission and goals of the educational institution and school of nursing are expressed most directly in the strategic plan. This plan must be given considerable attention. Outlining long and short-term goals, priorities, objectives, time-lines, and critical outcomes for the institution and school will give insights about institutional priorities achieved and yet to be achieved. Data from the strategic plan can lend support to or expedite proposed recommendations about curriculum. Conversely, knowledge of the strategic plan can signal potential roadblocks to curriculum development.

Culture

Organizations have a culture or a "way of being" that may not be directly evident. Organizational culture evolves over time and is slow to change. The culture is formed by determinants such as the people in the organization, how these people interact and make decisions, the endeavors and decisions pursued or avoided, and the consequences of these actions. A significant aspect of the culture is whether change is welcomed or avoided. If a new curriculum is premised on a changed culture in the school, curriculum developers must strategize carefully, since culture change is difficult to accomplish.

Financial Resources

Financial resources, possibly more than any other internal contextual factor, influence the curriculum design. Knowledge of the operating costs of a school, budget planning, and budget allocation is essential. Careful attention should be given to the cost created by a new or revised curriculum. The availability of adequate funding can constrain the curriculum design and is foundational to successful implementation. For example, it is better to know in advance that a particular teaching-learning strategy (such as a reliance on small-group learning) cannot be supported financially and to plan accordingly, than to develop a treasured curriculum and face the frustration and disappointment of learning that it is too costly to implement.

Programs and Policies

The programs and policies of the educational institution and the school of nursing form an important factor of the internal environment. Within the school, the type of programs, the number of programs, the physical and human resources dedicated to those programs, and the relationship of the developing curriculum to other programs will all influence curriculum design. For example, if health promotion is a strength of the graduate program, it would be reasonable to expect emphasis in this area in the new undergraduate curriculum.

The range of courses offered by other departments could either be an asset to the new nursing curriculum or limit its scope. Knowledge from the physical, biological, and psychosocial sciences, as well as from the arts and humanities, contributes significantly to nursing knowledge and well-rounded graduates. Availability of courses, pre-requisites, and scheduling should be ascertained, as well as the possibility of negotiating new support courses.

Curriculum development must be considered in light of existing policies and guidelines. Institutional and school policies and guidelines should be available to, and understood by, the curriculum development team. Changing school policies, as part of curriculum change, can be a complicated process and must be accomplished within the context of existing institutional regulations. Requests for policy changes that might affect the educational institution are more complex and can be expected to take a longer period of time to achieve.

Infrastructure

The term *infrastructure* refers to those elements that form the structure of the educational institution and school of nursing. These include human and physical resources, as well as resources to support teaching and learning. Data can be secured and scrutinized to obtain a comprehensive picture of the infrastructure.

Human Resources Human resources form the core of the curriculum and are the most important resources of the institution. According to Bevis (2000), "transactions and interactions that take place between students and teachers and among students [human resources] . . . are the curriculum" (p. 72). Indeed, as European universities were developing in the 10th and 11th centuries, professors and students [human resources] were the university and met wherever they could find space.

Faculty are key contributors to curriculum development and implementation, and represent a vital part of internal infrastructure. They are critical sources of insight and information about what to include in the curriculum, since they know what works, what doesn't, and why. They bring the curriculum to life, execute all its dimensions, and have a vested interest in student and program success.

Information about current nursing and non-nursing faculty and the pool of potential faculty is an important determinant of curriculum decisions. Additionally, adjunct faculty, guest lecturers, clinical experts, preceptors, and health care administrators form part of faculty resources. They need to be considered when shaping the curriculum, not only for the contributions they might make to the future curriculum, but also for the involvement and perspectives they can offer to curriculum development and implementation.

Students are an essential human resource. Schools of nursing would not exist were it not for students; without them, there is no need for curriculum. Student data form the basis of much internal contextual information critical to curriculum development. Changes in student characteristics could be instrumental in triggering curriculum changes. Table 5.1 lists student data that could be obtained to enhance understanding of the internal contextual environment.

Support staff represent other important human resources. Programs could not function without people such as secretaries, admissions officers, caretakers, information technology specialists, and others. They make possible the smooth day-to-day operations of the school. Gathering data about this group, such as numbers and skill sets, is mandatory.

Information about human resources includes details about contracts that govern the working life of faculty and staff. A review of faculty and staff collective agreements provides insights into matters such as job expectations, holiday entitlement, hours of work, and so forth. These all influence the curriculum. For example, if the educational institution were prohibited from assigning full-time faculty to teach on week-ends, then curriculum designers would have to weigh the educational value of week-end clinical experience for students against the effects of inaccessibility of full-time faculty.

Physical Resources   Availability and quality of materials and space for classrooms, offices, and laboratories must be considered. These must be sufficient to match the curriculum design and student learning needs. If curriculum developers are thinking of changing class size, they must first determine if suitable classrooms are available.

Technology (such as office computers, student computer labs, audio-visual and clinical equipment, smart classrooms, and distance technology) should be assessed. Technologies assist faculty to fulfill their roles efficiently, are necessary for effective teaching, and facilitate student learning.

TABLE 5.1   STUDENT DATA

Number of applicants

Number of admissions

Numbers meeting and exceeding admission requirements

Demographics:

- previous education
- age
- marital status
- number of dependents
- employment status

Catchment area

Proportion of full- and part-time students

Grade point average

Grades in nursing and support courses

Attrition rates and rationale

Success rate on national registration examinations

Follow-up data about graduates

- employment positions
- employer evaluations
- numbers admitted to graduate programs

Resources to Support Teaching and Learning   Resources that support teaching and learning should be examined. Knowing what is available within the school and institution will assist in making curriculum decisions, planning, and negotiating for additional resources.

Library resources are critical to enhance teaching and learning. Facilities and collections should be assessed to determine if they are sufficient to support the curriculum. A review of the library's holdings will identify the strengths and gaps in the library's collection. The availability of online databases has implications for curriculum and course designs, student assignments, and faculty research. Knowledge about shortcomings in library holdings provides a basis for negotiation for altered or expanded resources.

Faculty development services comprise another element of the internal infrastructure. School and institution-wide programs related to teaching and research development can be sources of ideas and support for the new curriculum. If, for example, institution-wide programs for developing online courses are provided, then curriculum developers will know that distance courses could be planned. However, if there are no programs relevant to teaching or evaluation in the new curriculum, then curriculum developers will have four choices:

- create and offer the faculty development program themselves
- hire a consultant
- negotiate for an institution-wide program that will not be specific to nursing
- avoid particular teaching and evaluation approaches in the new curriculum

Teaching support, such as graduate teaching assistants, or other university-employed or sponsored students, can extend faculty teaching. Typically, graduate students contribute to curriculum implementation through teaching, grading assignments, and leading tutorial sessions. Additionally, sources of funding for innovative teaching or curriculum, or for curriculum development, should be explored.

Student services related to assessment and development of academic skills, personal support, health, recreation, and financial assistance are integral aspects of the institutional infrastructure. These services can mean the difference between success and failure for many students.

An inventory of available resources, knowledge of future plans for resources and services, and the possibility of negotiating new plans, are influential when shaping and bringing vitality to the new curriculum. Curricularists must understand the infrastructure in which the new curriculum will operate so they can plan a feasible curriculum with conviction.

Summary of Internal Contextual Factors

In summary, internal contextual factors are those forces, situations, and circumstances that originate within the school and educational institution and have the potential to influence curriculum. These should be examined with two lenses. A macro lens captures the contextual data relevant to the institution; a micro lens focuses more specifically on the school of nursing.

External Contextual Factors

External contextual factors are those forces, situations, and circumstances that originate outside the educational institution and also have the potential to influence curriculum. They originate in the community, region, country, and world, that is, the environment beyond the educational institution.

Interestingly, as early as the 1970's, Conley (1973), urged curricularists to pay attention to social forces when planning or changing curricula. She referred to population mobility as one social factor in which persons are continually changing jobs, resulting in people lost on a medical landscape and becoming medically disengaged. She also cited the general sophistication of the public, a commercialization of the professions, wherein professionals are no longer altruistic but more interested in career ladders; and a change from a religio-philosophical orientation to a more scientific and research-based outlook. She observed the growth and spread of organized interest groups in the community, government, and unions, as well as in other organized conglomerates. Finally, she remarked on the shift in age composition and disease prevalence in the population. Her observations still hold true today, and are consistent with the external factors of relevance to current nursing curriculum developers.

An examination of external contextual factors is crucial to understanding the needs and characteristics of society and their application to contemporary nursing curricula. A brief survey of the most influential external contextual factors follows. Chapter 6 contains further examples of contextual data and how the data could affect the nursing curriculum.

Demographics

Demography is the systematic study of human populations and primarily addresses their growth, size, and infrastructure. Social demographers relate population data to the economics and culture of particular societies in different times and places to detect causes and influences of changing population trends (Reference Encyclopedia, 1998, p. 408).

Demographic data, which have a significant influence on health care delivery and nursing education, should be obtained. Information pertaining to population characteristics assists curriculum developers to know about the people who are and will be clients of the health care system. The nursing curriculum then can be designed to align with the attributes of those who are recipients of nursing care. Local, regional, and national data should be obtained. Pertinent census data and vital statistics include the following:

- birth, death, and fertility rates
- distribution according to age, sex, location, and combinations of these
- population diversity
- employment rates and income levels by age and sex
- ethnicity
- residence patterns (e.g., proportion of aged living alone, in nursing homes, etc.)
- morbidity rates and patterns
- family structures
- immigration and emigration patterns

Assessing population demographics is germane to developing relevant nursing curricula. Obviously, characteristics of human populations, i.e., the people nurses serve, which are gleaned from data outlining patterns of growth, migration, ethnic and racial composition, and health and illness, must be included in the repertoire of curricularists in order to construct a relevant curriculum.

Culture

Further to assessing the demographics of the human populations nurses serve, curriculum developers need to direct attention to the culture(s) within the external environment. Heightened cultural sensitivity will promote the development of a curriculum responsive to health care clients.

Culture refers to the ways of being of a particular group. Included in the concept are "a common history . . . shared sense of destiny, . . . distinctive language [with] an idiosyncratic vocabulary . . . a value order that is often embedded upon a particular cosmic design, religion, or mythology, . . . a distinct system of traditions and rituals, . . . narratives that give [express] norms, and models of behavior" (Sitelman & Sitelman, 2000, p. 12). This depiction of culture is extensive and captures many of the subtleties inherent in the individuals, groups, and communities that comprise the external environment in which the nursing program is situated.

There are many cultures within every community. Race and/or ethnicity are often equated with a particular culture (i.e., a particular set of practices, rituals, and beliefs), but this is not always the case. People of a particular ethnic origin may represent a unified subculture, or they may have been assimilated into the dominant culture. Additionally, each community has a number of subcultures which may not be immediately obvious, but which contribute to the tapestry of the community culture and, therefore, are relevant for curriculum planning. The cultures of poverty, family violence, homelessness, gender, aging, work environments, and the culture of the health care system are some examples.

Respect for the traditions, shared beliefs, values, attitudes, and norms of the distinctive cultures is advantageous when designing a curriculum. This is particularly important in the 21st century when cultural diversity is precipitated through immigration, emigration, and even technological advances linking individuals, groups, and communities within cyberspace.

Health Care

Demographics influence health care, another external factor relevant for curriculum planners. Pertinent information related to health, the health care system, and nursing education might include the following:

A. Health Care and Health Care System
- most prevalent local and national health problems
- nature of health care agencies and their services
- nature and availability of public health and other community-based health care services
- adequacy of funding for health care

- availability of health care insurance
- costs to clients and families
- availability of health care resources, i.e., health care services; equipment; health care providers; health educators
- profile of clients receiving care
- gaps in service

B. Nursing Education
- potential clinical placement sites
- receptiveness of clinical agencies to students
- willingness of health care providers to participate in student education
- opportunities for multi-, inter-, and trans-disciplinary health professional clinical education

Curriculum developers ought to gather data pertaining to varied educational settings for student clinical experiences, as well as data about the changes in health care problems, care services, and facilities. Furthermore, they need to be current about health care delivery patterns, escalating costs, and available resources. Additionally, they should be mindful of the needs and demands of more sophisticated health care consumers.

Professional Standards and Trends

Health care and nursing education standards affect the practice and education of nurses. Accordingly, nursing practice and education standards and trends influence curriculum development. Data to obtain include the following:

- position statements from professional organizations, nursing leaders and experts, administrators, researchers, graduates, and the public
- professional, regulatory, licensing, and accreditation requirements
- entry-to-practice, nursing practice, legal, and ethical standards
- self-assessment and quality assurance guidelines or requirements
- implementation of evidence-based practice
- research on nursing education and practice
- contemporary nursing education models, frameworks, philosophies, and teaching and learning approaches
- current and future roles and the scope of practice that nurses will assume

Technology

Advances in technology influence the content and teaching and learning strategies of the new nursing curriculum. Curricularists should gather data about the use of technology in health care and education. The information age, with access to computer technology has "re-shaped society . . . revolutionized life . . . changed the pace and possibilities in communication . . . [and has] multiple implications for nursing practice and education" (Rains Warner, 2005, p. 112).

> *It is imperative . . . that nursing education address the learning needs of students and prepare them to practice in the next millennium of health care. Mastery of information technology and managing health information are essential areas of curriculum content for all undergraduate and graduate nursing programs* (Carty & Philip, 2001, p. 405).

With this in mind, the curriculum development team needs to gather data about the technologies in use, and those expected to be used, so that they can prepare students for current and future practice.

Environment

Environmental data, which curriculum developers should examine, will most likely pertain to the developers' immediate community. However, because we live in a "shrinking" world, chemical, biological, physical, sociological, and psychological hazards and stressors can pose a health risk to local, national, and international populations. Accordingly, these are possible threats to individual, family, and community health and therefore, are important data for curriculum planning. These data could include some or all of the issues listed below, in particular those that seem most relevant to the locale of the school of nursing:

- weather patterns such as severe blizzards, extremely hot summers, tornadoes, or hurricanes
- climate changes
- air and water quality
- presence of local industries known to produce environmental pollutants and hazards
- environmental disasters, such as oil spills, volcanoes, forest fires
- decreased energy supplies
- nuclear and chemical spillage and warfare
- bioterrorism
- international spread of diseases, e.g., Sudden Acute Respiratory Syndrome (SARS), mad cow disease (bovine spongiform encephalitis), Avian flu, West Nile virus

Environmental health hazards, perhaps neglected heretofore, should be given attention when data-gathering for the envisioned nursing curriculum.

Socio-Politico-Economics

The contextual factor, *socio-politico-economics*, refers to social, political, and economic forces or issues in the external environment that have the potential to influence the new curriculum. This is a broad-based factor, since social, political, and economic events and issues are strongly interconnected, each affecting the others. For this reason, *socio-politico-economics* is presented as one contextual factor.

After data are gathered about the previously-identified external contextual factors (demographics, culture, health care system, professional standards and trends, technology, and environment), it is possible to discern their relationship to socio-politico-economics. However, there could be additional information about the context in which the curriculum will be operationalized. Examples are provided below.

A. Social issues that affect health can include:
  • drug use in the community
  • sexual behavior of adolescents
  • unemployment rates and patterns
  • housing availability, affordability, and quality
  • nature and rate of crime in the community

B. Political and legislative (local, regional, provincial/state, and national) influences, which affect:
  • higher education and nursing education
  • health care and social services
  • eligibility for health care and social services
  • support for nursing and nursing education from elected political parties, government officials, and community representatives
  • public concern about nursing shortages and access to health care
  • projections for a comprehensive health care system

C. Economic conditions, such as:
  • governmental financial support for higher education and nursing education
  • private, community, or public funding for:
    • curriculum innovation
    • program development

- faculty and student grants or scholarships
- present and projected local, provincial/state, and national economies

Curriculum stakeholders should carefully assess these and other social, political, and economic issues which can have a direct bearing on the envisioned curriculum.

Summary of External Contextual Factors

In summary, nursing curriculum developers must carefully consider those external contextual factors that can influence nursing practice and education. The curriculum must be responsive to demographic trends; culture; health care reforms; economic characteristics; nursing practice and educational standards; technological advances; political forces; transformed structure and needs of families and communities; links among knowledge, information, creativity, and wealth; globalization of the economy; and environmental fragility; in essence, those broad interrelated, complex and ever-changing socio-politico-economic influences that affect every aspect of our existence. Curricularists should be acutely aware of external contextual factors and how they impact the direction and pattern of nursing curricula. They cannot be oblivious to these forces, but must respond decisively, and design a bold curriculum that will be relevant now and in the future. The challenge is to prepare professional nurses capable of caring for culturally diverse individuals, families, and groups within a dynamic society and health care system.

Approaches to Gathering Data for Curriculum Development

Agreement about the contextual factors requiring investigation is followed by decisions about which data will be relevant, the sources of data, and the methods to obtain the information. The data gathering activities represent a strong public statement that a redesigned curriculum will be forthcoming. Gathering data is dependent on interactions between nursing faculty and other members of the educational institution, key personnel in health care agencies, and members of the community. Although the intention to change the curriculum is known to stakeholders involved in the planning that precedes data gathering, it is at this time that expectations for curriculum change are raised in the wider community. Because of the public nature of the data gathering activities, curriculum developers are obligated to present themselves in a credible manner. This requires planning and organization.

Deciding on Necessary Data and Data Sources

The quality and scope of data gathering about contextual factors, and the subsequent interpretation of the data, are foundational to the nature, relevance, and longevity of the curriculum.

When deciding on the data to be collected, data sources, and methods for gathering data, curricularists must strive to achieve a reasonable balance between a desire to acquire a breadth and depth of data on the one hand, and a need to progress in a timely manner on the other.

The required data must be agreed upon so that suitable sources can be identified and, if necessary, data gathering tools developed. There should be openness to the acquisition of data that is not initially identified but subsequently recognized as important. For example, it might be decided that data about the intended programmatic directions of the major health care agencies in the community would be essential, that particular heath care leaders are appropriate data sources, and that interviews would be the most expedient method of acquiring the data. If, in the course of an interview, an administrator comments that in order to introduce new programs, key clinical units will be closed for renovations, it would be prudent to ask for more information immediately, since there are clear implications for the curriculum. In making decisions about which data to collect, curriculum developers could consider the following:

- Contextual factors most relevant to the school of nursing.
  - Which contextual factors seem most germane to our situation?
  - What are the precise data we require?
- Potential utility of the data for the curriculum development process.
  - Which data will truly influence the curriculum?
  - What is "nice to know," but not absolutely imperative for curriculum development?
  - How might the data we have identified influence our curriculum?
- Accessibility and availability of the data.
  - How quickly can we obtain the data?
  - Is acquisition of any data so important that a delay in curriculum development is justified?
  - What are the consequences of failing to collect these data?

When deciding upon the necessary data for each of the contextual factors, the interrelated nature of the factors will be apparent: information gathered could be pertinent to more than one factor. It is best to obtain and record them for each factor, rather than debating where they belong.

A host of individuals, groups, organizations, and documents can be used as data sources to provide information that may influence curriculum decisions. Determining which sources would be most useful is dependent on the situation within each school of nursing. Criteria that guide these decisions include:

- richness of data likely to be obtained
- accessibility and availability of data sources
- purpose of data gathering (solely as a basis for curriculum development or also for research)
- resources available (time, people, finances, materials)

Methods of Gathering Data

Knowledge that shapes the curriculum is generally not collected according to the rigorous standards of research. However, attention must be given to the research approval and procedures if research is being conducted along with curriculum development. If there is overlap or ambiguity about what is research and what is simply information gathering, it is imperative that institutional definitions of research and policies about collecting information are heeded.

Many methods could be employed to gather data about internal and external contextual factors. Those that will yield valuable data as expeditiously as possible, and for which the curriculum designers possess the required skills, should be used. The most common methods of data gathering for the curriculum development process are reviewed below.

Literature Reviews and Internet Searches Ideas about current trends, philosophical approaches, and strategies for nursing education, along with significant directions for health care, can be acquired from literature reviews and internet searches. Learning about the convictions and opinions of experts, and the current state of nursing education beyond the local situation, will expand the perspectives of those involved in curriculum development and provide a national and international context for curriculum development. Ideas from beyond national borders often furnish new and relevant insights, even though the origins of the concepts or the implementation are geographically, and perhaps politically, distant. More specifically, published curriculum designs and examples of courses can serve as models for new curricula, while many authors offer suggestions that arise from the successes and difficulties they have experienced with curriculum design and implementation. Particularly valuable can be research reports about the effects of specific instructional strategies. These provide evidence that can guide future educational practices. Authors whose ideas particularly appeal to curriculum stakeholders can also serve as consultants at appropriate times during the curriculum and faculty development processes.

A critical analysis of nursing literature can provide insights into the ideological and political realities of nursing life and nursing education. Explication of these realities, as well as the values implicit in nursing literature (Masterson, 1998) can expand understanding of the nature and culture of nursing practice and education, and therefore, influence the nursing curriculum.

Document Review A review of existing documents can be an inexpensive means of acquiring data identified as necessary to the curriculum development process. Some documents may be readily available, such as professional practice and educational program accreditation standards, or the institutional mission, vision, philosophy, and strategic plan. Conversely, others may require a more protracted effort to obtain. These might include government or clinical agency reports. Those documents that are judged to have particular relevance for future curriculum directions should be reviewed and pertinent data extracted.

Key Informant Interviews Interviews (face-to-face, telephone, or email) can be an effective and inexpensive method to acquire pertinent data quickly. Plan the interview questions carefully so that maximum relevant information is acquired without unduly imposing upon the informant's time. It is imperative to record the responses (usually by note-taking) so that information is not forgotten. As the interview is ending, it is wise to confirm that it would be acceptable to follow up, either in person, by telephone, or email, if clarification or additional data are required.

Focus Group Interviews These are planned discussions intended to obtain information about a specified topic in a non-threatening environment. The group typically comprises 6 to 12 individuals with a common set of interests. A facilitator whose role is to assist the group to explore the topic in depth, generally within a loose structure, guides their discussion. Although the structure is not fixed, open-ended questions are prepared in advance. According to Krueger and Casey (2000), questions should be developed to match the following sequence of categories: opening, introductory, transition, key, and ending. Ideas are recorded (often on flipcharts in addition to audio-taping) and periodically reviewed to ensure accuracy of recording and comprehension. The goal is not consensus; rather it is a full exploration of the topic.

Halloran and Grimes (1995) describe their use of focus group methodology to generate data about what nurses need to know to care for persons with HIV and appropriate educational processes for a continuing education program. Similarly, a focus group of stakeholders (e.g., staff nurses, clinical educators, or clients) could provide input into a school's curriculum development process.

Surveys Face-to-face, telephone, mail, or email surveys are used to obtain data from a large number of people in a relatively short period of time. Questionnaires require time to construct so that the items are understandable to respondents and data can be readily analyzed. Examples of how surveys might be used in curriculum development include determination of opinions about health care and curriculum directions, views about the strengths and limitations of the current program and its graduates, information about the nature of nursing practice, and attitudes of nurses with graduate degrees toward future employment as faculty.

Delphi Technique Delphi technique is a survey forecasting tool that provides a means of obtaining input relatively quickly from stakeholders who may be geographically distant, but whose ideas are deemed essential. A panel of experts is asked to complete a series of questionnaires that address their opinions, judgment, or predictions about a particular topic (Polit & Beck, 2004). Each set of responses is summarized and another questionnaire sent to the same individuals for confirmation. The iterative process is repeated until consensus is achieved (Jairath & Weinstein, 1994).

The Delphi technique was used by five schools in British Columbia as they developed a collaborative nursing curriculum. To acquire the views of practicing nurses, they asked, "Given the changes that you have seen in your practice, what do you anticipate the nurse of the future will need to do, know, and be [in order] to provide high quality nursing care?" (Beddome et al., 1995, p. 12). From the responses, a questionnaire was developed, and after two rounds of responses, consensus was achieved about the 10 top-ranked items.

Consultations Consultations with experts and/or peers at other institutions can provide valuable knowledge, insights, and guidance about particular aspects of the curriculum (such as current philosophical approaches), future directions for nursing practice, and implementation challenges of particular curricular designs. Frequently, the counsel they offer is gained from experience that has not yet been committed to publication. The contributions of consultants and peers from other institutions can be substantial, but subsequently must be considered within local realities. Cost is likely a factor, and therefore, when a consultant is employed, it is wise to ensure that the purpose of the consultation has been explicated and as many stakeholders as possible are able to participate in the discussions.

Deciding on Data Gathering Methods When deciding on appropriate methods to gather data about the internal and external contextual factors, ask the following questions:

- What are the time and expertise we have for gathering data?
- What is the most expedient way to obtain the required data?
- What are the resources we have for developing data gathering tools and analyzing data?
- Do we have the necessary resources to employ the preferred data gathering methods?

The Work of Gathering Data

There is no formula for deciding which data to collect about the contextual factors, data sources to contact, and data gathering methods to employ. Rather, curriculum developers should give attention to the questions and considerations posed in the sections above. Then, using their knowledge of the school, their experience, and their judgment, they can reach consensus about what is reasonable and realistic. The conclusions will likely be different for each school. A work sheet could help focus thinking about data gathering and, when posted, serve as a visual reminder of work to be completed.

Table 5.2 presents examples of data, data sources, and data gathering methods for the internal contextual factors of philosophy, mission, and goals; culture; financial resources; and infrastructure. Table 5.3 presents similar information about the external factors of culture, health care systems, and professional standards and trends.

TABLE 5.2 EXAMPLES OF DATA, DATA SOURCES, AND DATA GATHERING METHODS FOR INTERNAL CONTEXTUAL FACTORS

Internal Contextual Factors	Data	Data Sources	Data Gathering Methods
Philosophy, Mission, and Goals	Published philosophy, mission, goals, strategic plan	Institutional and school documents, websites	Document review
	Values and guiding principles	Key informants, e.g., senior academics, current and former faculty, school dean or director	Interviews
Culture	People	Organizational charts	Document review
	Interaction styles	Key informants, e.g., senior academics, chair of institutional planning committee, administrators	Interviews
	Decision-making and processes (formal and informal)		
	Aspirations		
	Values		
	Openness to change		
	Relationship with other organizations		
Financial Resources	Priorities for institutional budget	Institutional planning documents	Document review
	School budget (current and projected)	Key informants, e.g., senior academics and administrators, faculty, staff	Interviews

continues

TABLE 5.2 CONTINUED

Internal Contextual Factors	Data	Data Sources	Data Gathering Methods
	Projected budget for curriculum planning and implementation	School of Nursing dean or director	Document review
Infrastructure *Human resources*	Employment agreements	Collective agreements	
	Nursing Faculty		
	Number of part- and full-time	School of Nursing dean or director	Interviews
	Credentials and expertise	Faculty	
	Expected retirements and resignations		
	Characteristics of adjunct faculty		
	Pool of potential faculty	Chairs of graduate programs	Interviews, surveys
	Pool of potential clinical preceptors	Clinical agencies	Survey, focus groups
	Non-Nursing Faculty		
	Availability and interest of non-nursing faculty to teach (and possibly develop new) support courses	Department Chairs	Interviews

continues

	Students		
	Characteristics and number of applicants	Registrar, Chair of school admissions committee	Interviews
	Demographics of current students	Admissions committee reports	Document review
	Attrition and completion rates	School records	
	Support Staff		
	Numbers	School of Nursing dean or director	Interview
	Skill sets		
Physical resources	Office space	Physical plant documents	Document review
	Classroom space and facilities		Observation
	Labs		
	Technology	Information technology group	Interviews
	Library		
	Nature of holdings	Library staff	Interviews
	Computerized resources	Listing of current holdings	Document review
	Faculty Development Services		
Resources to support teaching and learning	Nature and availability of services	Director of institution-wide services	Interviews
	Possibility of creating new services	School of Nursing dean or director	Document review
		Published information (print- and web-based)	Web search

99

TABLE 5.2   CONTINUED

Internal Contextual Factors	Data	Data Sources	Data Gathering Methods
Teaching support			
	Availability of graduate teaching assistants	Program chairs School of Nursing dean or director	Interviews
	Access to institutional funding	Funding announcements	Web search
Student Services			
	Nature and availability of services	Director of student services	Interviews
	Possibility of creating new services if warranted by changed curriculum	Published information (print- and Web-based)	Document review

TABLE 5.3   EXAMPLES OF DATA, DATA SOURCES, AND DATA GATHERING METHODS FOR EXTERNAL CONTEXTUAL FACTORS

External Contextual Factors	Data	Data Sources	Data Gathering Methods
Culture	Values, beliefs, and practices of dominant culture	Key informants of ethnic, cultural groups	Interviews
	Ethnic and groups in community	Publications of major ethnic and cultural organizations	Document review
	Values, beliefs, and practices of subcultures		
	Values, beliefs, and practices of health care system and providers	Mission statements of health care agencies	Document review
		Published codes of ethics, political positions of professional organizations	
Health Care	Services provided by hospitals, community health agencies, and private providers	Promotional materials, websites, agency leaders	Document review, Web search
	Plans for changes in health care services	Health care executives, leaders	Interviews
	Identified gaps in service	Government policy statements	Document review, Web search
	Sources of health care payments	Local or provincial/state reports (print or web-based)	
	Ratio of registered to non-registered staff in major agencies	Annual reports, human resource personnel	Document review, interview

continues

TABLE 5.3 CONTINUED

External Contextual Factors	Data	Data Sources	Data Gathering Methods
	Receptiveness of nursing staff to students	Nursing staff	Interviews
		Nursing executives	Survey, focus groups
Professional Standards and Trends	Practice regulations	Licensing and accrediting bodies	Document and Web site review
	Licensure requirements	Professional bodies	Document review
	Scope of practice requirements and restrictions	Legislation	Document review
	Nursing care priorities and trends	Professional bodies, literature, practicing nurses	Document review, focus groups
	Professional ethics and ethical issues		Delphi technique
	Approval and accreditation standards	Approval and accrediting bodies	Literature and Web searches
	Nursing education trends	Nursing education leaders, literature, and internet resources	Survey, interviews
	Teaching-learning models	Experts (peers and consultants)	Interviews
Socio-politico-economics	Government policies and regulations	Government reports (written and web-based)	Document review, Web search
	Institutional, local, national and international policies		
	Public finances		

Grants, scholarships, and other funding for students, faculty, and school	Alumni associations, professional bodies, foundations	Document review, Web search
Political support for nursing education	Newspapers, government and political reports	Web search, document review
	Influential community and political representatives	Interviews
Public messages about nursing and nursing education by nursing leaders	Publications by professional organizations	Document review, Web search
	Nursing leaders	Interviews

The work of gathering data may be given to a task force or shared more widely among stakeholders. Sufficient time should be allowed for this aspect of the curriculum development process to ensure that a full picture is obtained of the internal and external contexts. If the new curriculum is to endure for approximately a decade, it must be based upon accurate and comprehensive data.

It is helpful to have a central repository for the data so that it will be readily accessible for subsequent analysis. Additionally, methods that will speed up analysis (such as immediate computer entry of returned questionnaire responses by a secretary or research assistant) should be employed whenever possible.

During the phase of data gathering, ideas will arise about possible curriculum directions. It is natural to begin to think about how particular data could influence the curriculum. Record these ideas, but remember that they are only tentative possibilities, based on incomplete knowledge. However tempting it may be, try to avoid drawing premature conclusions from partial data about what the curriculum should be like. It is only when all data are assembled, interpreted, and synthesized that well-founded curriculum directions will emerge (see Chapter 6).

Faculty Development

The overall goal of faculty development in relation to gathering data about contextual factors is to expand members' appreciation and knowledge of the influence of these factors on curriculum development. Faculty development can include a session in which internal and external contextual factors are reviewed. Discussion about which factors are significant and how these factors can influence curriculum development will help novice curriculum developers understand the need for systematic data gathering. During such a discussion, some pertinent data, data sources, and data gathering methods can be identified, with details being reserved for a task force or committee

Likely, some attention will need to be given to differentiating between gathering data for curriculum development and data collection for research. It may be appropriate to include information about, and practice in, interviewing key informants if this will be a new activity for some. These faculty development activities can be readily facilitated by those members with expertise in data gathering and curriculum development.

Chapter Summary

Gathering data about internal and external contextual factors, which have the potential to influence curriculum directions, is a public activity that heralds a forthcoming curriculum change. Stakeholders must first identify those factors that are most relevant to the school of nursing and curriculum development. Then, decisions must be made about pertinent data, data sources, and methods. Adequate time must be given to gathering this information, since the strength and longevity of the new curriculum will rest upon the quality of the data gathering and the subsequent analysis. Faculty development prepares members for the decisions and activities that comprise data gathering about contextual factors.

Synthesis Activities

Below are two case studies. The Poplarfield University School of Nursing case will be continued in Chapter 6, where the data provided below will contribute to the determination of curriculum directions. Consider the critique of the case and whether additional ideas merit discussion. The second case is followed by questions to guide examination of the case. Questions to determine faculty readiness for gathering data conclude this section of the chapter.

Poplarfield University School of Nursing

Poplarfield University is a 50-year-old institution that began as a federally-funded agricultural college to support the farming community that surrounds the town. The college was located in this rural area to provide direct assistance to farmers by agricultural experts, opportunities for local higher education, and a site for crop research relevant to the area. Over time, the focus of the institution expanded to include forestry, science, arts, and 15 years ago, nursing. The intent was that local students prepared in nursing would remain in the community after graduation.

Poplarfield is a town of 60,000 people, largely supported by the farming economy and by a military base approximately 10 miles away. The original stands of poplar trees have given way to family farms and large agri-business operations.

The 85-bed Poplarfield Hospital provides emergency care, non-critical in-patient care, and rehabilitation. Ambulatory services support in-hospital care. Critically ill individuals are sent to a large medical center 100 miles away. The local public health unit has a mandate to provide health promotion and maintenance programs to individuals, families, and communities. The University provides non-emergency health services for students; the military offers the same type of health care to its members and their families. Two occupational health nurses are responsible for the work-related health concerns of the employees of a large meatpacking plant.

The School of Nursing offers two undergraduate programs: a 4-year BSN program (total enrollment 150) and a post-RN degree completion program. Enrollment in the latter program increased markedly 6 years ago when baccalaureate entry-to-practice was mandated, but applications have been down to only 10–12 for each of the past 2 years. All classroom courses in the school of nursing are taught by 10 masters-prepared faculty, while most clinical teaching is conducted by baccalaureate-prepared faculty.

The original nursing faculty were members of the Poplarfield Hospital School of Nursing, which closed as the university program began. The two remaining original faculty members will retire within the next 2 years. Other faculty have been recruited, generally directly out of master's programs. They tend to stay for 2 or 3 years and then leave the community. Only the director, Dr. Mary Werstiuk, has a PhD, and she is expected to remain at the school as long as her husband continues his university appointment.

Under Dr. Werstiuk's leadership, the faculty are undertaking curriculum development. A consultant has helped them to understand the influence of contextual factors on the curriculum, curb their tendency to make premature decisions about the new curriculum, and plan their data gathering activities. They have decided that the most important external contextual factors are demographics of the community and the nursing workforce, the health care needs and resources of the community; and competing institutions and programs. They intend to review the mission, priorities, resources, and policies of the university and school. Careful attention was given to identifying data sources, methods of obtaining the data, and individuals to complete the tasks. They have given themselves three weeks for gathering contextual data.

Critique The faculty of Poplarfield School of Nursing have taken important steps to be systematic and focused in their data gathering activities. They have identified important contextual factors, data sources, methods of obtaining the data, and individuals to undertake the work. It is necessary for them, however, to be precise about which data are important and to match data gathering methods with the type and sources of desired data.

For example, when considering demographics, the faculty are correct in being concerned about the profile of people in the community. They need to specify that they are interested in knowing the age profile, the birth and death rates, whether young and elderly people typically stay in the area or move elsewhere, the rate of immigration, etc. Past and current information of this type can be obtained from government agencies responsible for tracking the population. By defining and obtaining the desired information, faculty will develop a picture of the community that subsequently will allow them to make inferences about potential students and health-care clients. The faculty need to be equally diligent in specifying the data for each of the contextual factors they have identified.

Faculty would be wise to consider other contextual factors, such as professional and accreditation standards. These, along with trends in nursing education, are essential for faculty to know as they develop the curriculum to ensure that the new curriculum will conform with required standards and will either be in line with or ahead of current curriculum thinking.

Similarly, faculty should review the full range of internal contextual factors and relevant data. For example, when assessing human resources, they need to determine why nursing faculty stay for only 2 or 3 years. Within the university, strategies to attract and retain faculty, as well as retention patterns, would be valuable information to acquire.

Members of the Poplarfield University School of Nursing should further consider their plans for data gathering. They need to review the contextual factors and determine which others are relevant to them. Then, they need to define the data about each factor that could be of value to curriculum development, ascertain the appropriate sources, and specify the best means to obtain the data from those sources. Data collection will likely extend beyond 3 weeks. Incomplete data collection will eventually hamper curriculum design, and faculty will have to return to this aspect of the curriculum development process.

Bellemore University School of Nursing

Bellemore University, an accredited, long-standing institution of some 150 years, with approximately 10,000 full- and part-time students, is located in a mid-western industrial city of 350,000 inhabitants. University departments offer programs in liberal arts, social, physical, and health sciences. The four-year baccalaureate-nursing program is one of three others within Health Sciences. Eighty students are admitted annually to the nursing program, which has a total complement of 300 students in the four years. The majority is female and enrolled on a full-time basis. Approximately 25% of students study part-time, are mature, and have taken jobs in the community in order to meet tuition costs.

Thirty full- and part-time faculty, 15 with doctoral degrees, 12 with masters preparation, and 3 with baccalaureate degrees teach classroom and clinical courses in the school of nursing. The nursing program received full accreditation 4 years previously.

The main industry of the city of Bellemore, for which the university is named, is automobile manufacture. The largest auto plant, which employs approximately 2000 workers, offers health services to all employees.

In addition to the university, the city of Bellemore boasts a 3000-student technological community college, as well as the following health facilities and services: a 450-bed acute care general hospital; a 275-bed long term and chronic care facility; 3 physician-serviced medical clinics; 2 walk-in emergency clinics; and a county community health department.

Bellemore School of Nursing is preparing for a change in its four-year baccalaureate program. The need to examine the contextual factors that will affect nursing practice, and hence the curriculum in the next 10–15 years, is recognized as important to designing a future-oriented, relevant curriculum.

Dr. Amèlie Le Blanc, the curriculum coordinator, requested a meeting of curriculum representatives from faculty, students, and community health personnel, to discuss contextual factors relevant to a redesigned curriculum. The group decided to schedule a faculty development session to help them with this activity. As a result of this session, several task force groups were formed to determine who would participate, which relevant data would need to be gathered, the sources, methods, and tools for this undertaking. The group agreed to meet again when the contextual data gathering phase was complete.

Questions for Consideration and Analysis of Bellemore University Case

1. Which contextual factors would be most relevant to Bellemore's vision of a future-oriented nursing curriculum?
2. What are the essential data to collect about these contextual factors?
3. Which data gathering methods and tools might be employed to obtain information about the contextual factors?
4. What would be a suitable time period for collecting and collating these data?
5. Who could best participate in this data gathering activity? How could they organize to obtain relevant data expeditiously?

Curriculum Development Activities for Consideration in Your Setting

The questions below will assist in determining readiness for gathering data in your setting.

1. Which are the internal and external contextual factors that we deem important?
2. What are the precise data we need to obtain about each factor?
3. What (or who) are the best sources from which to obtain the data?
4. How should we proceed to obtain the data?
5. Who is available to gather the necessary data?
6. What resources do we have available to prepare data gathering tools and to analyze data?
7. How do we ensure there is sufficient time for gathering data?
8. What location can we use as a central repository for data?
9. What faculty development activities might best prepare us for gathering data?

References

Beddome, G., Budgen, C., Hills, M., Lindsey, A.E., Manchester Duval, P., & Szalay, L. (1995). Education and practice collaboration: A strategy for curriculum development. *Journal of Nursing Education, 34*, 11–15.

Bevis, E.O. (2000). Nursing education as professional education: some underlying theoretical issues. In E.O. Bevis & J. Watson (Eds.), *Toward a caring curriculum. A new pedagogy for nursing* (pp. 67–106). Boston: Jones and Bartlett Publishers.

Carty, B., & Philip, E. (2001). The nursing curriculum in the information age. In V. Saba & K. McCormick (Eds.), *Essentials of computers for nurses: Informatics for the new millennium* (3rd ed.) (pp. 393–412). New York: McGraw-Hill.

Conley, V.C. (1973). *Curriculum and instruction in nursing.* Boston: Little, Brown and Company.

Halloran, J.P., & Grimes, D.E. (1995). Application of the focus group methodology to educational program development. *Qualitative Health Research, 5,* 444–453.

Jairath, N., & Weinstein, J. (1994). The delphi methodology (part one): A useful administrative approach. *Canadian Journal of Nursing Administration, 29*–42.

Kreuger, R.A., & Casey, M.A. (2000). Focus groups: A practical guide for applied research, 3rd ed. Newbury Park, CA: Sage Publications.

Masterson, A. (1998). Discourse analysis: A tool for change in nursing policy, practice & research. In P. Smith (Ed.). *Nursing research: Setting new agendas* (pp. 81–107). London: Arnold.

Reference Encyclopedia. (1998). Oxford NY: Oxford University Press.

Polit, D.F., & Beck, C.T. (2004). *Nursing research: Principles and methods* (7th ed.). Philadelphia: Lippincott.

Rains Warner, J. (2005). Forces and issues influencing curriculum development. In D.M. Billings & J.A. Halstead (Eds.), *Teaching in nursing: A guide for faculty* (2nd ed.) (pp. 109–124). St. Louis: Elsevier Saunders.

Sitelman, F.G., & Sitelman, R. (2000). Ethics and culture: From the claim that God is dead, it does not follow that everything is permitted. In M.L. Kelley & V.M. Fitzsimons (Eds.). *Understanding cultural diversity: Culture, curriculum and community in nursing* (pp. 11–21). Sudbury, MA: Jones and Bartlett.

CHAPTER 6

From Contextual Data to Curriculum Directions and Outcomes

Chapter Overview

Once data-gathering about internal and external contextual factors is complete, and the data assembled, it is time to integrate the information and determine its meaning for the curriculum.

Following a definition of terms used in this chapter and explicit to this book, is a description of the cognitive processes involved in the analysis, interpretation and synthesis of contextual data. These include integrating data, inferring curriculum concepts and professional competencies that a nurse would require, proposing curriculum possibilities, deducing curriculum limitations, and identifying administrative issues that affect curriculum design. Also discussed are syntheses of the ideas generated from the contextual data collectively, and how they lead to curriculum directions and outcomes. To enhance clarity, the thinking processes that bridge data-gathering and the emerging curriculum directions and outcomes are presented in a procedural fashion. However, the processes are iterative and integrative in nature, with all ideas influencing previous and subsequent thinking.

As in other chapters, faculty development activities are suggested. After the summary, an extended case illustrates the main ideas. Questions to guide analysis are included, as well as questions to stimulate thinking about developing curriculum directions and outcomes in individual settings.

Chapter Goals

- Appreciate the multiple cognitive processes inherent in analysis and synthesis of contextual data

- Recognize how internal and external contextual data influence curriculum directions and outcomes

- Consider faculty development activities related to analysis, interpretation and synthesis of contextual data and the development of curriculum directions and outcomes

- Examine an account of a hypothetical school's development of curriculum directions and outcomes

Definition of Terms

A number of terms are introduced which are presented in a conceptually logical order, rather than in a more conventional alphabetical sequence:

Curriculum concepts are abstract ideas that form the substance of the curriculum.

Professional competencies are the abilities required for nursing practice. These include, but are not limited to, cognitive, affective, technical, and interpersonal skills, as well as the integration and judicious use of these skills within the context of nursing. Knowledge is prerequisite to all professional competencies. Examples of professional competencies might include:

- cognitive: problem-solving, critical thinking, clinical reasoning
- affective: caring, respect, professional values and ethics
- technical: health-care procedures and technologies, information technologies
- interpersonal: communication, relationships, leadership, supervision

Curriculum possibilities are imaginative ideas about teaching-learning experiences, curriculum design options, and potential content areas.

Curriculum limitations are restrictions or constraints on teaching-learning experiences, curriculum design options, or potential content areas.

Administrative issues are those logistical, personnel, and/or budgetary matters which are beyond the authority of faculty members to resolve, but which can significantly affect the new curriculum.

Curriculum directions are conclusions about curriculum concepts, teaching and learning processes, and design options drawn from the synthesis of the contextual data, curriculum concepts, curriculum possibilities and limitations, and administrative issues. They are the basis of subsequent decision-making about the curriculum.

Curriculum outcomes refer to the synthesis of professional competencies, derived from the analysis, interpretation, and synthesis of contextual data.

Analysis, Interpretation, and Synthesis of Contextual Data

Analysis (determining essential elements), interpretation (deriving meaning), and synthesis (combining parts to form a whole) of the contextual data to arrive at curriculum directions and outcomes are iterative and interactive processes that require reflective thought, an open mind, and free communication. Despite the fact that these are clearly non-linear, in this chapter they are deliberately presented separately. This should facilitate explanation and understanding of curriculum processes that might not have been explicated previously. It should also make apparent the relationships among contextual data, curriculum directions, and curriculum outcomes.

Analyzing data about contextual factors and deriving meaning to reach conclusions about curriculum directions and outcomes entail a confluence of examination, integration, interpretation, reflection, and inference-making about curriculum concepts and professional competencies: generation of curriculum possibilities and limitations, identification of administrative issues, and decision-making. These deliberations occur in collaboration with colleagues whose perspectives, conclusions, and values may be divergent.

Five processes are described as part of the analysis, interpretation, and synthesis of contextual data. They are:

1. examining and integrating contextual data; identifying patterns and trends
2. inferring curriculum concepts and professional competencies
3. proposing curriculum possibilities
4. deducing curriculum limitations
5. identifying administrative issues

Although presented separately, these processes occur almost in tandem since ideas about the new curriculum are generated through free-flowing discussion. Ideas relevant to all aspects of the process arise concurrently, with one thought sparking many others.

Examining and Integrating Contextual Data

Examining and integrating data is an activity for the Total Faculty Group (see Chapter 3). All those who develop and eventually implement a new curriculum must understand the context in which the curriculum will be operationalized and in which graduates will work. Individual members should review the data about the contextual factors, determine the influence factors have upon one another, and generate ideas about trends. This individual review becomes the basis for discussion by the Total Faculty Group. Collectively, members discuss the ideas that were generated individually and identify patterns or trends. Data, patterns, and/or trends will reveal the current "state of affairs" and form the basis of a relevant curriculum. Curriculum developers can ask:

- What data are available about this factor?
- What patterns and/or trends emerge from the data?

Review and discussion about data and trends for individual factors will make apparent the overlap and connections among contextual data for several factors, and how data and trends about one contextual factor will influence and be influenced by data and trends of other factors. The overall goal of reviewing contextual data and identifying trends is to achieve an integrated view of the data and a shared understanding of the "big picture" of the context in which the curriculum will be operationalized and graduates employed. The questions that might be considered are:

- How do data or trends about one particular factor affect trends in other contextual factors? For example, how could changing funding for health care affect the health of an aging population?
- If these or any other trends continue, what might that mean for other contextual factors? For instance, what might declining fertility rates mean for public health programs related to parental-child health?
- What are the dominant features of the context in which graduates will be employed?

Predicting possible futures in response to these questions helps curriculum developers anticipate the context for which the curriculum will be developed and in which it will be implemented. In understanding the "big picture," curricularists also come to agreement about which contextual factors should be *most important* in determining curriculum directions and outcomes. *More important* factors may be readily apparent and agreed upon; *less important* might require discussion and consensus. There is no need to reach quantitative conclusions about the relative importance of each factor. Instead, faculty members need to reach accord about the comparative weight of all contextual factors so that the *most, more, and less important* ones are determined. In this way, the curriculum becomes responsive to the predominant influences.

Inferring Curriculum Concepts and Professional Competencies

Review of contextual data, trends, and patterns will lead to insights about curriculum concepts, abstract ideas that form the substance of the curriculum. As well, professional competencies essential for nursing practice can be inferred. The professional competencies, as noted previously, include but are not limited to cognitive, affective, technical, and interpersonal skills, as well as integration and judicious use of these skills.

Curriculum concepts and professional competencies are inferred mainly from the external contextual factors, although some may also be evident from internal factors. As well, further ideas are stimulated about these curriculum concepts and professional competencies by those already suggested. The generation of these ideas occurs concurrently, not sequentially. Curriculum developers can ask:

- What inferences about important curriculum concepts, those that students will need to know and apply in nursing practice, can be made from the contextual data and from patterns and trends?
- What inferences about professional competencies can be made from the contextual data, from patterns and trends, and from curriculum concepts?
- What additional ideas about relevant curriculum concepts arise from the professional competencies that have been suggested?
- What additional ideas about professional competencies arise from the curriculum concepts that have been suggested?

The intent is to list all the ideas that arise from brainstorming, without concern about the format in which they are expressed.

Proposing Curriculum Possibilities

From ideas about curriculum concepts and professional competencies, thoughts about curriculum possibilities flow spontaneously. Curriculum possibilities (i.e., imaginative ideas about teaching and learning experiences, curriculum design options, and potential content areas) result from creative thinking, unfettered by consideration of logistics. To determine the curriculum possibilities of the contextual data, curriculum concepts, and professional competencies, ask the following:

- What possibilities arise from the contextual data, patterns, trends, curriculum concepts, and professional competencies about:
  - teaching and learning processes and experiences?
  - curriculum design options?
  - potential content areas?

Ideas about curriculum possibilities can be drawn directly from data, trends, curriculum concepts, professional competencies, or from a combination of these. If, for instance, the majority of faculty has educational and experiential credentials in community health, then it will be evident that a community-focused curriculum is possible. If, as another example, the curriculum concept of *professional responsibility* and the competencies of *critical thinking* and *political action* are determined, then experience with the political action committee of a professional organization might be proposed as a curriculum possibility.

The goal is to generate many ideas about curriculum possibilities. Some may seem "off the wall" and others more conventional. The apparently outlandish possibilities may be appealing, but impractical. However, with subsequent application of pragmatic and logical thinking, these might be modified into innovative and feasible suggestions.

Inferences about curriculum concepts and proposals about curriculum possibilities could lead to considerable discussion and debate, even when only a single contextual factor is being examined. For instance, some faculty may interpret a low fertility rate in the community as signaling a need for a curricular emphasis on prenatal assessment and health promotion, while others may conclude that maternal-infant health requires little attention. Some ideas may fit more than one category, and debate could arise about this, an example being health promotion seen as professional competency, concept, and potential content area. Repeated recording of the same idea in several categories likely signifies its importance.

It is useful to record all thoughts that occur, and at this stage to avoid debate about suitability, categorization, inclusions, or exclusions. Such decisions will be made in subsequent integrative discussions about curriculum directions and outcomes, and curriculum and course design (see Chapters 8 and 9). The reason for producing and recording as many ideas as possible is that they naturally arise from an examination of the contextual data and help curriculum developers move toward curriculum directions and outcomes. Remember, however, that the ideas being recorded are tentative, and will likely be modified as curriculum development proceeds.

Identifying Curriculum Limitations

In contrast to curriculum possibilities, curriculum limitations are restrictions or constraints on teaching and learning experiences, curriculum design options, or potential content areas. These are derived from a pragmatic or logical interpretation of the contextual data, trends and patterns, curriculum concepts, professional competencies, and curriculum possibilities. Curriculum builders need to ask:

- How do contextual data and trends constrain what might be possible in the curriculum?
- What restrictions do curriculum concepts and/or professional competencies place on curriculum possibilities?

Both internal and external contextual data can point to curriculum limitations that warrant serious attention by the curriculum team. For example, a faculty group whose clinical expertise lies mainly in acute care might identify the faculty profile as a limitation if community-based clinical experiences have been proposed as a curriculum possibility. Another example could be that particular clinical experiences are constrained by limited availability of student placements.

Importantly, some of the curriculum possibilities and limitations can lead to actions that could profoundly change the school and the curriculum. For example, data about the nursing profession would likely include a statement describing the current and projected worldwide shortages of nursing faculty. This fact could limit the likelihood of successfully implementing a small-group, case-based curriculum, which would require relatively large numbers of faculty. Alternately, it could spur faculty to lobby senior administrators to initiate vigorous faculty recruitment and retention efforts.

Deducing Administrative Issues

Invariably, administrative issues that might affect the curriculum will become apparent as contextual data are analyzed and curriculum possibilities and limitations identified. Administrative issues, those logistical, personnel, and/or budgetary matters that are beyond the authority of faculty members to resolve, can significantly affect the new curriculum. The question to be answered is: *What logistical, personnel, and/or budgetary issues should be raised with the school leader?*

It is worthwhile to note administrative issues and bring them to the attention of the dean or director, specifying the effects they could have on the curriculum and stating the desired resolution. Then, with the school leader's support and leadership, strategies can be developed to address the issues. Indeed, curriculum design will likely be dependent on the resolution of some matters. Curriculum developers and school leaders must take the necessary steps to address the administrative issues, including securing resources required for the future curriculum.

Summary of Processes

Several processes have been described to illuminate the thinking that emanates from the contextual data: examining and integrating contextual data, inferring curriculum concepts and professional competencies, proposing curriculum possibilities, identifying curriculum limitations, and deducing administrative issues. Although delineated separately, the processes are interactive and occur almost concurrently, each idea influencing others.

Table 6.1 presents an example of the conceptual links that exist between data and curriculum for the external contextual factor of *Demographics* for the Poplarfield case from Chapter 5. Included is an abbreviated set of contextual data, and the patterns and trends arising from the data. Curriculum concepts, professional competencies, curriculum possibilities and limitations, and administrative issues are suggested. The columns in the table provide a convenient and organized method of recording ideas, but are not meant to connote sequential thinking.

TABLE 6.1 EXAMPLE OF CONCEPTUAL LINKS BETWEEN CONTEXTUAL DATA AND CURRICULUM FOR POPLARFIELD UNIVERSITY SCHOOL OF NURSING

External Contextual Factors	Data	Patterns and Trends	Curriculum Concepts	Professional Competencies	Curriculum Possibilities (P) and Limitations (L)	Administrative Issues
Demographics	**National** Fertility rate inadequate to sustain population (1.52 children/woman)	Decline in fertility rate Fewer births Reduced proportion of infants and children in the population		Maternal-infant care	**P:** Increased or decreased maternal-infant health **L:** Reduced opportunities for maternal-infant clinical experiences	
	Life expectancy = 81.7 years for women; 76.3 for men Largest proportion of population born between 1946–64 (baby boomers)	Increasing numbers and proportion of seniors; seniors will be the largest population group	Nursing care and health promotion of aging population	Care of elderly in homes and community facilities Managing resources	**P:** Clinical experiences in homes; long-term care facilities; inpatient, outpatient, and community settings **P:** Continuum of care from hospital to home	Preparation of faculty for community-focused care Development of new clinical sites
	Increasing numbers of the very old	Improved health into old age, coupled with increased numbers of those with acute and chronic illness		Health maintenance and promotion throughout the life span	**P:** Nursing in primary, secondary, and tertiary care settings	New clinical practice sites

Population growth through immigration, mainly from mid-East, Eastern Europe, Southeast Asia, Africa, Caribbean	Cultural diversity of recipients of nursing care	Nursing care of those with chronic illness	**P:** Child & adult development
	Countries of origin changing from Western Europe to more global pattern	Culturally and ethnically sensitive nursing care Cultural competency Assessment throughout the life span Communication Critical thinking	**P:** Theoretical or conceptual framework for planning and delivering nursing to individuals of varying cultural beliefs and practices **P:** Approaches to health maintenance and promotion that build on traditions of immigrants
Poplarfield area: Birth rate = 1.16 children/woman Proportion of 20–40 year olds decreasing, as they migrate to cities	Lower than national rate Numbers of infants and young children will decrease as adults of child-bearing and -rearing age decrease Pre-conception, prenatal, and perinatal health of both parents Assessment, health promotion		**L:** Pre-, intra-, and post-natal clinical experiences
Retired farmers generally move into the town of Poplarfield	Social and health consequences of lifestyle changes		**P:** Urban and rural clinical experiences Travel difficulties for many students

continues

TABLE 6.1 CONTINUED

External Contextual Factors				Curriculum Possibilities (P) and	Administrative
Data	Patterns and Trends	Curriculum Concepts	Professional Competencies	Limitations (L)	Issues
Immigration into town of Poplarfield mainly from Philippines, India	Changing ethnic heritage of Poplarfield residents	Cultural competency	Cultural competency	**P:** Home visiting to expand students' understanding of cultural and ethnic influences on health and illness	
Seasonal farm workers from Mexico, most of whom do not speak English and do not have health insurance; present from early June to October each year.		Values Culture	Responding to health care needs of short-term local residents, for whom cost is a factor Nursing care of marginalized groups Identification of own values, biases	**P:** Rural clinical experiences to address the health needs of migrant workers, urgent care clinics, street nursing	Contracts and insurance for student experience in non-traditional sites
Large numbers of young adults at local armed forces base		Promotion of life-long health habits during young adult years	Health promotion	**P:** Clinical experiences on armed forces base **P:** Health promotion with members of armed forces	Development of new clinical sites

Determining Curriculum Directions and Outcomes

The integrated view of all the contextual data, patterns and trends, provides curricularists with a holistic impression of the internal and external environments of the school of nursing. This understanding is required to plan a curriculum relevant to the context in which it will be implemented and in which graduates will work. Synthesis of curriculum concepts, possibilities, limitations, and administrative issues leads to curriculum directions, such as teaching and learning processes and curricular design options. Synthesis of professional competencies should result in the curriculum outcomes. Below is a suggested process for determining curriculum directions.

First, the curriculum concepts proposed from the *most important* contextual factors are reviewed, and commonalities are integrated. Then, the same process is followed separately for the *more important* and *less important* contextual factors. The three sets of curriculum concepts that emerge are synthesized, with attention to the factors' relative importance. Any concepts not yet integrated are re-examined to ensure that relevant ones are not omitted. The synthesized concepts become part of the curriculum directions.

There may be agreement to delete some concepts, or it might seem more suitable to leave that decision to later when more detailed curriculum planning occurs. Questions to guide the synthesis of the curriculum concepts are suggested in Table 6.2.

When synthesizing curriculum possibilities and limitations, the same process is followed. The teaching and learning processes and design options that emerge should be assessed

---

TABLE 6.2   QUESTIONS TO GUIDE SYNTHESIS OF CURRICULUM CONCEPTS

- What are the commonalities among curriculum concepts inferred from **each** of the *most important, more important,* and *less important* contextual factors?

- Can curriculum concepts inferred from the *more* and *less important* contextual factors be integrated with those from the *most important* contextual factors?

- Of those curriculum concepts that have not been integrated, which should be included in the curriculum?

- Does the synthesis reflect the relative weighting assigned to the contextual factors?

- Are there ideas, evident from the combination and inter-relationships of contextual factors, that have not been identified?

- Does the synthesis truly encapsulate the important ideas that are essential for graduates to know and use, so they can practice successfully in the health care system of the next decade?

within the realities of administrative issues. The agreed-upon teaching and learning processes and design options become part of the curriculum directions, along with the synthesized concepts.

Professional competencies identified for each factor are synthesized in the same fashion. The synthesized competencies become the curriculum outcomes. Similar questions to those proposed in Table 6.2 could be used to determine curriculum outcomes.

Although potential content areas and specific learning experiences may have been suggested as part of the curriculum possibilities, detailed attention is not given to these now. Rather, the ideas are retained for future review and consideration, when curriculum design and detailed course planning occur.

Finally, the curriculum team must employ its judgment about the curriculum directions and outcomes that have been determined. Members will want to review all the work that has been done. Questions to consider include:

- Are curriculum directions and outcomes really appropriate for the context?
- Has anything important been missed?
- Are there other curriculum directions or outcomes that should be discussed?
- Are the curriculum directions and outcomes congruent with the developing philosophical approaches? (See Chapter 7)
- Can faculty collectively support the directions and outcomes that have been stated?

To reach agreement about curriculum directions and outcomes, considerable discussion could be necessary. Understandably, decisions can be fraught with conflict if aspects of the current curriculum valued by particular faculty members are likely to be excluded or reduced in prominence. It is natural for faculty to use the current curriculum and personal teaching experience as a frame of reference for discussion. If a consensus is difficult to reach, it would be wise to review the reasons for curriculum redesign, the data about the most important contextual factors, and values held by faculty. This re-examination could lend objectivity to the discussion.

The Total Faculty Group must achieve resolution about curriculum directions and outcomes. Agreement is essential, because a successful curriculum is dependent on total support. Final decisions about curriculum directions and outcomes should be clearly justifiable by the constellation of contextual data, and responsive to the reasons that led to curriculum development in the first place. Only then can curriculum developers be assured that they are developing a curriculum that will be relevant in the future. From decisions about curriculum directions and outcomes, goals are formulated (see Chapter 7), and details of curriculum design flow (see Chapter 8).

Faculty Development

The goal of faculty development in relation to analysis, interpretation, and synthesis of contextual data is to expand appreciation and understanding of the processes involved in deriving curriculum directions and outcomes from contextual data. Participants require a thorough understanding of these processes since decisions about curriculum directions and outcomes will shape the school for a number of years. After the contextual data-gathering is complete, a development session overviewing analysis, interpretation, and synthesis of the data would be helpful.

Faculty development, in workshop format, can be focused on the processes that will move faculty and other stakeholders from contextual data to curriculum directions and outcomes. First, participants could discuss the contextual data to gain a common understanding of the environment. Then, they might divide into groups to derive curriculum concepts, professional competencies, curriculum possibilities and limitations, and administrative issues for one contextual factor. In this way, all could have experience in the analysis of the same contextual factor, so that differing perspectives would be evident. Alternatively, the remaining contextual factors could be divided among groups, with each to consider a different factor, thereby expediting the curriculum development process. Practice with the processes leads to understanding. In both approaches, presentation of the subgroups' work could lead to values clarification, and further discussion about the process of deriving curriculum directions and outcomes. Faculty development activities can be facilitated by those members with experience in this aspect of curriculum development, or if appropriate, by an outside expert.

Chapter Summary

In this chapter, a further step in the curriculum development process is described, namely the interpretation and synthesis of contextual data to derive curriculum directions and outcomes. The processes of analyzing, interpreting and synthesizing the contextual data are emphasized as being iterative and non-linear, although a procedural approach is described for explanatory purposes. Questions are provided to assist in integrating data, inferring curriculum concepts and professional competencies, proposing curriculum possibilities, identifying curriculum limitations, and deducing administrative issues. Determining curriculum directions and outcomes, and discussing inclusion or exclusion of particular curriculum concepts and possibilities, involve emotions and values. Therefore, open communication, values clarification, and rigorous intellectual discussion are essential to achieve an informed analysis and synthesis of contextual data and the formulation of future-oriented curriculum directions and outcomes. Faculty development activities are key in preparing participants for this work.

Synthesis Activities

The Poplarfield University School of Nursing case is continued from Chapter 5 with faculty and other stakeholders now developing their curriculum directions and outcomes. This extended case includes tables to illustrate how contextual data can be analyzed. For purposes of brevity, not all data are presented. The intent is to demonstrate the development of curriculum directions and outcomes. Questions are provided for analysis of the case.

Because of the length and complexity of the Poplarfield University School of Nursing case, a second case for analysis is not included. The chapter concludes with questions to guide the development of curriculum outcomes and directions relevant to your school of nursing.

Poplarfield University School of Nursing

Members of the Poplarfield University School of Nursing completed their data-gathering about internal and external contextual factors. A curriculum consultant was hired for a two-day retreat to help the group derive curriculum directions and outcomes from the data. Dr. Werstiuk, the School Director, stated her intention to attend and participate fully. The Dean of the Faculty was also invited, since her support would be needed for any additional resources that might be required for the new curriculum. Faculty believed that her involvement would be an effective means to educate her about the complexity of curriculum planning and the multiple factors which influence nursing programs. Additionally, members of the Curriculum Advisory Committee were invited to attend, and two of the twelve members were able to do so.

In preparation for the retreat, the data had been organized for each factor and a hard copy distributed to all faculty, using the chart that faculty had agreed would be useful. A copy of the chart was loaded onto laptop computers, so that ideas could be immediately recorded and preserved.

The group agreed to derive the curriculum directions and outcomes collectively, starting with a shared understanding of the environment. They were committed to the ideas of inferring curriculum concepts and professional competencies, proposing curriculum possibilities, and deducing curriculum limitations. There was consensus to dismiss identification of administrative issues, since "we already know what the issues are: not enough faculty and not enough money in the budget."

Examining and Integrating Contextual Data During the course of discussion about contextual data, the faculty tried to focus on the meaning of the data, and the inter-relationships among the contextual factors. They also addressed curriculum concepts, professional competencies, and curriculum possibilities without labeling these ideas as such, discussing ideas about how:

- the presence of more aged people leads to a greater demand for health care, which increases the requirement for health care professionals
- the growing RN shortage could increase public demand for more seats in nursing programs, and this in turn would necessitate more resources for the School, including human resources
- RN shortages could lead to more care by nonprofessionals, increasing the need for RNs to delegate and supervise. The RN shortage might result in specialization by all RNs or de-professionalization of nursing
- computer-competent students could be developed in a school where faculty have limited expertise with computer-mediated learning
- professional standards for nursing practice, accreditation standards, and the availability of clinical placements in and near Poplarfield can be reconciled
- local health problems can be addressed, in a society and health care systems which are focused on problems of national scope, such as cancer
- nursing priorities and mandates must be explicated for a society with a growing proportion of old people and a health care system where acute care stays are shortened and out-of-hospital care is increased

The group also talked in detail about some specific data. For example, when examining the external contextual factor of *Demographics*, faculty members began to debate the meaning of the low birth rate in the community, with some faculty convinced that poor maternal health was a factor. They believed that an emphasis on preconception and prenatal health would be essential in the curriculum. Others asserted that the low birth rate is simply a reflection of a societal trend toward smaller families. The group decided to accept, for now, that there were divergent views about that data.

In trying to reach a shared understanding of the environment in which the curriculum would be implemented and graduates would work, several integrated summaries were offered. Each resulted in some disagreement. Finally, at the end of the morning, the group agreed that the environment could be described as one in which:

- there will be less institutionalized health care and growing emphasis on community-based care
- independent decision-making and supervision of non-professional health care providers will become a stronger feature of nursing practice

- vulnerable groups in the community may grow in size
- the proportion of aged people in the community will increase, while young people will continue to leave the Poplarfield area
- ethnic diversity will become more apparent
- agriculture will continue to be a significant economic factor in Poplarfield

In the afternoon, discussion progressed to identification of the factors that should be most influential in shaping the curriculum. Initially, there was a strong sentiment that all contextual factors were of equal weight, apart from the internal factors of *History; Philosophy, Mission, and Goals; and Culture,* all of which seemed less important. The consultant agreed that the factors are highly inter-connected and that the division of the data into these factors is somewhat artificial. Yet, she reminded faculty that there must be some basis for identifying the major curriculum influences, and thus for determining the curriculum outcomes and directions.

The group then considered whether it was the recipients of nursing services (*Demographics*), the nature of nursing (*Professional Standards and Trends*), or the location and nature of health care (*Health Care*) that was most important. Faculty phrased this as *who, what, where* and *how*. Finally, they agreed that most important were the people being served, and therefore, *Demographics* and *External Culture* would be most significant in determining curriculum directions. *History* was immediately labeled as being of least importance. They concurred that *Health Care, Professional Standards and Trends,* and the school's *Infrastructure* would all be second in importance, followed by *Socio-politico-economics*, and then *Technology*. *Environment; Philosophy, Mission, and Goals;* and *Internal Culture* were deemed to be of approximately the same importance as *History*. This was summarized simply by listing the contextual factors in rank order:

1. Demographics; External Culture
2. Health Care; Professional Standards and Trends; Infrastructure
3. Socio-politico-economics
4. Technology
5. Environment; Philosophy, Mission, and Goals; Internal Culture; History

Inferring Curriculum Concepts and Professional Competencies, Proposing Curriculum Possibilities, and Deducing Curriculum Limitations The stakeholders wanted to complete this intellectual work together, in the belief that it was necessary for everyone to participate in every aspect. Ideas were recorded on charts, which had been loaded onto their laptop computers.

It became apparent that one more day would be insufficient to complete this work, if the group continued in the same way. The consultant suggested that the contextual factors might be divided among smaller groups and the group agreed to think about this proposal.

The next morning a member of the Advisory Committee proposed that working in small groups would expedite the curriculum work. There was now consensus about this. Three smaller groups were formed and each took responsibility for some of the internal and external factors.

In reviewing the contextual data, members recognized that curriculum concepts, professional competencies, and curriculum possibilities and limitations did not necessarily arise from each internal factor. However, they noted that the data about some of the factors could ultimately influence decisions about curriculum, either limiting or propelling the curriculum design. For example, when examining the School's infrastructure, they recognized that the existence of computer labs for students meant that computer-based learning was a possibility, whereas the School budget and faculty numbers could constrain the curriculum. Accordingly, they reaffirmed their intention to identify the curriculum possibilities and limitations as they examined each contextual factor. As the groups worked, they recognized again that the contextual factors do not operate in isolation and that their ideas reflected the inter-related nature of the environment. The ideas arising from the internal and external contextual data were recorded.

Initially, questions arose about ideas that were offered. For example, when reviewing data about the history of the university and school, one faculty member suggested that the university and school history could form a potential content area and that comparison of the current and the new curriculum was possible. Some faculty disagreed, and others did not understand this proposal. Considerable discussion ensued. Finally, one member suggested that they record ideas, reserving evaluation.

Identifying Administrative Issues   Moreover, as they worked, they quickly recognized that there were administrative issues beyond faculty numbers and budget. Accordingly, the groups considered and recorded the administrative issues. They also recognized that *Financial Resources* was an important contextual factor.

At the end of their two days together, the participants felt proud of their work. All were eager to proceed with synthesis of the completed work, and the determination of curriculum outcomes and directions. See Table 6.1 for analysis of the external contextual factor of *Demographics*. Table 6.3 presents the internal factors of *Financial Resources* and *Infrastructure*. Table 6.4 outlines the analysis of the external factors of *Culture, Health Care,* and *Professional Standards and Trends.*

Determining Curriculum Outcomes and Directions   Resources were not available for an additional retreat day. Therefore, the group agreed:

TABLE 6.3 CONCEPTUAL LINKS BETWEEN INTERNAL CONTEXTUAL DATA AND CURRICULUM FOR POPLARFIELD UNIVERSITY SCHOOL OF NURSING

Internal Contextual Factors	Data	Patterns and Trends	Curriculum Concepts	Professional Competencies	Curriculum Possibilities (P) and Limitations (L)	Administrative Issues
Financial Resources	University budget is dependent on government funding	Prevailing feeling that inadequate budgets constrain activities				Additional funding required from senior administrators
	School budget meets salary and daily operational costs for current curriculum		Budgeting	Financial management in nursing practice	L: Curriculum design affected by budget	Investigation of new funding sources
	Discretionary funds range from none to "almost none"	Tight budget for many years with no extras				
	No travel funds for faculty				L: Introduction of more expensive teaching approaches	Travel funds necessary to renew, recruit, and retain faculty
					L: Purchase of learning resources	
					L: Faculty exposure to nursing education trends through literature only	
	Small budget for annual faculty development day					
	Budget secured from senior administrators for curriculum development				L: Faculty development to support new curriculum	Sufficient funds required for ongoing faculty development

Infra-structure a) *Human resources*	*University*		
	Retention of new post-doctoral faculty a concern across campus	Strategies in place in other schools to attract and retain faculty	**P:** Part of curriculum development budget for faculty development
	School of Agriculture has highest faculty retention rate among all schools: low teaching loads, extensive research funding, university's sole graduate program		**L:** Recruitment and retention of nursing faculty problematic
	All other schools have travel funds to support conference attendance		**L:** Few full-time, continuing faculty to develop and implement a high-calibre, rigorous curriculum
			Need for senior administrators to support strategies for nursing faculty recruitment and retention

continues

TABLE 6.3 CONTINUED

Internal Contextual Factors	Data	Patterns and Trends	Curriculum Concepts	Professional Competencies	Curriculum Possibilities (P) and Limitations (L)	Administrative Issues
School Faculty:	Director is PhD-prepared				**L:** Non-researchers may be unable to incorporate research into curriculum	Circular success dependent on adequate numbers of PhD, full-time, permanent faculty
	8 full-time, masters prepared; 2 to retire within 2 years	School has been unable to attract PhD faculty or retain full-time faculty			**L:** Curriculum developers may not be present for implementation	Need to attract and retain PhD faculty
	New full-time faculty receive 2–3 year contract; stay only 2–3 years, leave for larger cities				**L:** Many who will implement curriculum are not involved in its development	Faculty profile will affect accreditation
	15–22 part-time per term, baccalaureate prepared; approx. $\frac{1}{2}$ work part-time because of family responsibilities; others are	Relatively stable group of part-time faculty				Need to orient part-time faculty to new curriculum Investigate possibility of converting some

also employed elsewhere				part-time positions to full-time
Students				
BSN program: 80% from Poplarfield area; remainder from rural areas; 95% directly from secondary school	Student population is mainly local and rural	Rural health	**P:** Eliminate Post-RN program	Possibility of recruiting more students
Post-RN students: from Poplarfield and surrounding area	Decreasing interest in Post-RN program		**P:** Revitalize Post-RN program with adult learning approaches, accelerated model	Resources to support adult learning approaches
Staff				
3 full-time secretaries with roots in the community; all skilled in office computer applications	Stable group of support staff			Retain staff
b) *Physical resources*				
School has adequate space for current needs			**L:** Size, number, and configuration of classrooms limit increase in class size or seminar groups	Improved and expanded physical space required
Nursing building in need of refurbishing; updating				
Up-to-date computers for faculty and staff	University ensures that technology is current		**P:** Increased reliance on computer-based learning	Faculty preparation for alternate learning

continues

TABLE 6.3   CONTINUED

Internal Contextual Factors	Data	Patterns and Trends	Curriculum Concepts	Professional Competencies	Curriculum Possibilities (P) and Limitations (L)	Administrative Issues
					P: Computer-based courses	teaching modalities essential
c) *Resources to support teaching and learning*	*Library resources* Wide range of nursing texts and practice journals Few nursing research journals				L: Curriculum devoid of research base for nursing practice and nursing education	Necessary to expand research journals and texts
	Faculty development services One faculty member appointed full-time to assist with faculty development across campus				P: Assistance with alternate teaching and learning approaches	
	Nursing faculty have informal mentoring system for new full-time faculty	Continuous mentoring required				Formal mentoring necessary for faculty retention Need for ongoing faculty development

Faculty development re: new teaching and evaluation approaches

Information technology

Computer literacy

P: Rigorous curriculum

P: Computer-based learning

Resources available to help students be successful

Orientation program re: clinical teaching and evaluation for all new full- and part-time faculty

Student services

Computer lab open 18 hrs each day

Academic and personal counseling

Health services

Financial aid services

TABLE 6.4 CONCEPTUAL LINKS BETWEEN EXTERNAL CONTEXTUAL DATA AND CURRICULUM FOR POPLARFIELD UNIVERSITY OF NURSING

External Contextual Factors	Data	Patterns and Trends	Curriculum Concepts	Professional Competencies	Curriculum Possibilities (P) and Limitations (L)	Administrative Issues
Culture	Multicultural town No local ethnic radio or TV stations No ethnic restaurants	Dominant culture is North American, with some families retaining elements of culture of origin (e.g., special foods)	Cultural norms, values, and traditions	Cultural assessment Cultural competence Family assessment	**P:** Support course related to culture	Faculty development Negotiation for support course
	Farming community values nature, land, independence, yet always ready to help others	Farm women isolated		Health promotion Assessment of social relationships Provision of support	**P:** Clinical experiences with farm families	Transportation for students
	Immigrant adults from Philippines and India largely maintain own ethnic traditions and religious practices; children caught between cultures	Over past 5 years, more Filipino and East Indian applicants to nursing program	Intercultural stress	Empathy Effective communication with diverse groups	**P:** Health promotion and care of isolated individuals and groups	Access to ethnic groups

Seasonal workers from Mexico do not speak English	Seasonal workers are "outsiders"	Marginalization	Health care of disadvantaged groups	**P:** Clinical practices with immigrant and community groups	Access for clinical experience
Military personnel value discipline, order	Social distance and distrust between officers and enlisted personnel		Health promotion Critical thinking	**P:** Clinical experiences with immigrant and community groups	Access for clinical experience
Many younger military personnel socialize in Poplarfield bars on weekends	Increased number of bar brawls in past 2 years				
Drug use considered acceptable by approximately $1/3$ of young adults	Rise in use of "recreational drugs" Change in student culture	Responding appropriately in situations of values conflict Nurses' potential to make a difference	Assessment and intervention re: drug use Self-reflection Critical thinking	**P:** Clinical experiences in schools, drug rehabilitation centers, street clinics	Awareness of policies re: drug use Potential value conflict between faculty and students
Health Care Health care insurance available Rising costs of health care	Shorter hospital stays; higher patient acuity; more community- and home-based care to contain costs; greater burden of care on families	Health care system Community-based care	Assessment Resource management Independent decision-making Political astuteness	**P:** Home- and community-based care **P:** Analysis of health care system	

continues

TABLE 6.4   CONTINUED

External Contextual Factors	Data	Patterns and Trends	Curriculum Concepts	Professional Competencies	Curriculum Possibilities (P) and Limitations (L)	Administrative Issues
	Migrant workers generally do not have health insurance		Marginalization Equity Health care for those uninsured	Cultural competency for care to those who do not have health insurance	**P:** Health care for uninsured	
	Primary health care provided by family physicians, nurse practitioners, and public health units	Less in-hospital care in Poplarfield and surrounding area			**P:** Clinical experiences in physicians' offices, walk-in clinics, nurse practitioners	
	Secondary health care provided by Poplarfield Hospital; tertiary care and cancer treatment center 100 miles away	Shorter hospital stays; sicker people at home; home nursing care; increasing burden of care on family	Community-based care Health promotion Effective health care teams	Health promotion of individuals, families, communities	**P:** Emphasis on community-based and outpatient health promotion and acute nursing care	
	Shortened hospital stays			Community-based care throughout the life span and health-illness continuum		

Increased in-home nursing care required				
Increased acuity of hospitalized clients				
Many long-term care facilities in and near Poplarfield so residents can be close to home	Increasing numbers of 'old-old' in institutions	Care of permanently institutionalized, with a variety of care needs	Assessment of individuals and families	**P:** Clinical experiences in facilities for institutionalized elderly; residential care; mental health, in- and outpatient facilities	Access for clinical experience
		Psychological, social, and spiritual health, coupled with waning physical (and possibly cognitive) health	Family health promotion		
			Evidence-based practice		
			Critical thinking		
			Empathy		
			Information search skills		
Major health problems:					
Local incidence of coronary artery disease and most cancers consistent with national incidence	Determinants of health		Health promotion	**P:** Clinical experiences related to major health problems in acute, rehabilitation, and outpatient facilities	Negotiation re: clinical practice sites
	Genetics		Screening		
	Lifestyle		assessment, intervention		
	Heart health				
	Cancer care				

continues

TABLE 6.4   CONTINUED

External Contextual Factors	Data	Patterns and Trends	Curriculum Concepts	Professional Competencies	Curriculum Possibilities (P) and Limitations (L)	Administrative Issues
	High incidence of leukemia among older farmers—attributed to past unsafe use of fertilizers	Expected to continue for the next 20 years until that generation has died	Rural health Safety	Health assessment Safety counseling	**P:** Home visits to farms	Logistics of recruiting families for student visits
	Injury and accidental death of toddlers and young children on farms double the national incidence		Safety in agricultural environments Primary prevention Rural health	Screening assessment, intervention Screening assessment, intervention	**P:** Home visits to farms	
	Family violence recognized as a public health problem	Reporting has increased	Family violence Physical and emotional abuse	Screening assessment, intervention, referral related to family violence and abuse	**P:** Attention to signs of abuse and violence in all clinical settings	
	Nursing workforce: Average age = 46 years Average retirement age = 55 years	Nationwide shortage of registered nurses will worsen markedly	Provision of safe care despite workplace barriers	Maintenance of standards of excellence	**P:** Increase enrollment	Increased resources needed to increase enrollment

continues

		Recruitment and retention of nursing staff of concern	Leadership Supervision of, and delegation to, non-professional care-givers Critical thinking Information search skills Independent decision-making	Leadership, including supervision of, and delegation to, non-professional care-givers Team-building Creation of empowering workplaces Evidence-based practice Critical thinking	**P:** Leadership experiences, including supervision of non-professionals **L:** Fewer mentors and preceptors	Securing, orienting, and rewarding clinical preceptors
Professional Standards and Trends	Professional practice standards	Emphasis on accountability, critical thinking, evidence-based practice, professional development	Professional roles, responsibilities, accountabilities, standards Codes of ethics Critical thinking Evidence-based practice Professional development Inter- and multidisciplinary practice	Commitment to ethical standards, life-long learning Competent, ethical practice Inter-, multi-, and trans-disciplinary practice	**P:** Standards could drive curriculum design **P:** Standards and ethics in all courses **P:** Interdisciplinary courses, practice **P:** Research focus, evidence-based practice guidelines in all courses	Negotiating inter- and multidisciplinary courses

TABLE 6.4 CONTINUED

External Contextual Factors	Data	Patterns and Trends	Curriculum Concepts	Professional Competencies	Curriculum Possibilities (P) and Limitations (L)	Administrative Issues
	BSN degree required for all new entrants to nursing profession, beginning 2010 Competency-based registration examinations that are integrative, not based on medical model Non-university nursing programs closing or forming collaborative degree programs with universities	University preparation for all nursing students	Professionalization of nursing Nursing history Role of professional associations	All competencies of professional nursing	**P:** Increase in applicants to program **P:** Competency-based examinations **P:** Partnering with other educational institutions	Support for program expansion and collaboration with colleges Possible loss of some autonomy Need to determine views of senior administrators
	Program accreditation standards include: faculty research, inclusion of research focus in curriculum, link between clinical settings and curriculum			Research focus, evidence-based practice, best practice guidelines in all courses Reflective practice Self-directedness	**L:** Faculty are not researchers **L:** Library holdings scant in area of nursing research **P:** Research course	Hiring of PhD faculty and research development support Continuous assessment of program

Caring curriculum in vogue nation-wide Phenomenological curricula at some schools	Feminist, humanistic-educative approaches have supplanted behaviorist curricula	Nature of relationship with clients, colleagues	Critical thinking Respect Egalitarian rela-tionships	**P:** Concept-based teaching-learning **P:** Practice-driven curriculum **P:** Learner-designed assignments **L:** Faculty preparation and motivation	Time and cost of faculty development Faculty recruitment Supportive environment

- to distribute hard copies of the analysis of the contextual factors, so all could individually review the work that had been completed by all groups
- to use a regularly-scheduled faculty meeting to collectively review the work and add ideas that might have been omitted
- to reorganize individual schedules so they could meet from 3–7 PM twice in the next 2 weeks to determine curriculum directions and outcomes
- that Dr. Werstiuk and the Dean would meet to discuss the identified administrative issues, and plan further discussion with senior administrators, if necessary.

There was consensus that Professor Rose, Chair of the Curriculum Committee, would lead the discussions. As well, members were enthusiastic about the possibility of adding ideas to the work of other groups. Professor Rose asked that all try to ground their thinking in the work to date and, as much as possible, to look beyond personal beliefs.

The subsequent meetings were lively, and at times, tense. Review of curriculum concepts, professional competencies, curriculum possibilities and limitations, and administrative issues went quickly, with some additional ideas offered. There was a sense of accomplishment at the end of the first meeting, and impatience to get on with the definition of curriculum directions and outcomes.

At the first 4-hour meeting, there was consensus that synthesis of curriculum concepts, professional competencies, and curriculum possibilities should be completed collectively. Some important curriculum concepts were: *aging; health promotion; nursing care of people at home, in the community, and institutions;* and *nurse-client relationships.*

Professor Rose reminded them of the weighting they had assigned to the contextual factors, noting that they had not attended to all the factors they had weighted as second in importance. With this, the group returned to the *Health Care,* agreeing that the curriculum should address *local health problems* as well as *national* ones. In considering *Professional Standards and Trends,* faculty confirmed that a strong emphasis on *health promotion* was warranted, and agreed that *illness intervention* must be included. One member noted that *rural health* was an important concept that had been omitted, and there was immediate agreement to include it.

In synthesizing curriculum possibilities, the group decided that the important teaching and learning processes would be *self-direction, collaborative learning,* and *use of information technologies.* A more *contemporary curriculum design* would be created. Synthesis of professional competencies led to the conclusion that the most important curriculum outcomes would be: *critical thinking, clinical reasoning, independent and collaborative decision-making, cultural competence,* and *life-long learning.*

The group recognized that acceptance of these ideas would require resolution of administrative issues related to human, physical, and financial resources, along with faculty development. Dr. Werstiuk reaffirmed her commitment to work toward resolution of these matters.

The contentious discussion was about exclusions in the new curriculum. Tertiary care (a strong content area in the current curriculum) seemed not to be a priority. This was difficult for Professors Herme and McCarthy who were teaching this content, and at one point, they left the meeting, noticeably distressed. Dr. Werstiuk waited a few minutes, and then also left, intending to seek out her two colleagues and ask them to raise their concerns in the group. In talking with Professors Herme and McCarthy, she helped them summarize the reasons for curriculum change and, informally, clarify their values about the need for nurses who will be responsive to health care situations in the future. She acknowledged that she was concerned about how she herself would fit into the new curriculum, since her teaching was in traditional maternal-infant care and it seemed this would be diminished in prominence. She further stated that she believed the only way she could influence the new curriculum was by participating in its planning. Dr. Werstiuk invited Professors Herme and McCarthy to return to the session.

Silent for about half an hour following her return to the meeting, Professor Herme subsequently excited the group by asking them to consider a summer acute-care clinical experience in the city, a time when other nursing students would not be present in the facilities. Such an arrangement could move program completion forward by 4 months. Professor McCarthy extended the idea by suggesting that it might be possible to make this a co-operative service-learning experience, so that students would be paid a stipend by the agencies, while receiving educational supervision and academic credit from the university. Participants expressed appreciation to Professors Herme and McCarthy for thinking beyond the traditional program structure and agreed to give this idea full consideration as they proceeded with curriculum development.

The group felt satisfied with their curriculum directions and outcomes and confirmed they could support these ideas as the basis for subsequent curriculum development. Dr. Werstiuk and Professor Rose congratulated the participants on their hard work, creativity in reconciling varying perspectives, and intellectual courage in envisioning a curriculum that would require considerable change and learning by each member. All were proud of themselves individually and collectively, and anxious to begin the intensive planning that would bring their ideas to fruition.

Questions for Consideration and Analysis of the Poplarfield Case

1. What strengths and limitations are evident in the processes undertaken by the Poplarfield faculty? How might these processes be applied in other settings?

2. How might the retreat have been organized differently to advance the curriculum work?

3. Review Tables 6.1, 6.3, and 6.4. What gaps and overlaps are present in the contextual data?

4. Examine Tables 6.1, 6.3, and 6.4. Propose other interpretations of the data, major concepts, curriculum limitations and possibilities, and administrative issues.

5. Consider the curriculum directions and outcomes identified by the Poplarfield faculty. Do they seem reasonable? Could others be proposed?

6. What strategies could be implemented to keep the momentum going in the curriculum development process?

7. If you were to assume the role of curriculum consultant for the Poplarfield University School of Nursing, in what way might your actions be similar or different from those of Professor Rose?

Curriculum Development Questions for Consideration in Your Setting

Use the following questions to guide thinking about the development of curriculum directions and outcomes in your curriculum work.

1. How can the contextual data be organized and displayed in a manner that will be helpful for analysis?

2. What procedures could be used for analyzing, interpreting, and synthesizing the contextual data?

3. How can a common understanding of the contextual data be reached?

4. How can the relative weighting of the contextual factors be determined?

5. How can relevant administrative issues be deduced?

6. What procedures will lead to conclusions about curriculum directions and outcomes?

7. How can we be confident that the curriculum directions and outcomes are responsive to the reasons that led to curriculum development in the first place, and to the constellation of contextual data?

8. How might divergent viewpoints be addressed constructively?

9. What strategies can we employ to ensure that the identified curriculum directions and outcomes will be supported?

CHAPTER 7

Developing Philosophical Approaches and Formulating Curriculum Goals

Chapter Overview

In this chapter, philosophy is introduced with definitions and purposes. These are presented from the perspectives of general education and nursing education. Traditional philosophies are considered first, then some of the more current philosophies for nursing curricula, followed by the authors' conceptualization of philosophical approaches for curriculum development. It is not the intent of this section to present a detailed description of philosophies. Rather, they are synopsized to highlight main ideas, similarities and differences, and to stimulate pursuit of further understanding.

Subsequent to the section on philosophy, curriculum goals are described according to definition and purposes. Formulating curriculum goals follows. Then, faculty development related to philosophical approaches and curriculum goals, and a chapter summary are presented. Synthesis activities, including two cases, and questions for curriculum developers, conclude the chapter.

Chapter Goals

- Understand definitions and purposes of philosophical approaches and goals in curriculum development.

- Recognize the value of philosophical approaches and curriculum goals for the nursing curriculum.

- Consider processes for developing philosophical approaches and formulating curriculum goals.

- Reflect on faculty development activities related to developing philosophical approaches and formulating curriculum goals.

Curriculum Philosophy

Definition and Purpose of Philosophy

Philosophy is the "love and pursuit of wisdom by intellectual means and moral self-discipline . . . It comprises statements of enduring values and beliefs held by members of the discipline . . . Philosophical statements are practical guides for examining issues and clarifying priorities of the discipline" (Haynes, Boese, & Butcher, 2004, p. 77).

General Education   In general education, philosophy statements include assumptions about human nature, purpose and goals of education, instruction, students, learning, and roles of teachers, students, and programs. John Dewey, one of America's greatest educators, interpreted philosophy as a general theory of educating, whereas one of his students, Boyd Bode, viewed it as a source of reflective consideration. To Ralph Tyler (1949), a leader in curriculum development throughout much of the 20th century, philosophy defined the purpose of education, clarified objectives and learning activities, specified faculty roles, and guided the selection of learning methods and strategies. More recently, the view of philosophy is that it assists in making decisions for the profession (White & Brockett, 1987), in curriculum development (Wiles & Bondi, 2002), and in professional development (Petress, 2003).

Nursing Education   The traditional view of philosophy in nursing education is that the philosophy provides a value system that grounds the curriculum. It provides a basis for selecting and using curriculum concepts, theories, teaching methods, and learning experiences (Yura, 1974; Bevis, 1986; Marriner-Tomey, 1988; Clayton, 1989). It governs thought and conduct within a nursing program (Lawrence & Lawrence, 1983).

Gates (1990) proposes that a philosophy for nursing education should be open rather than hidden, and should profess the position of the nursing school and curriculum in the wider social context. In a somewhat different vein, Rentschler and Spegman (1996) suggest that the philosophy of the nursing profession is transmitted through a philosophy of education, and that students are socialized into the profession through the lived experience of nursing education.

Traditional views of philosophy prevail, and contain foundational values and beliefs for the nursing curriculum, teaching and learning (Dillard, Sitkberg, & Laidig, 2005; Csokasy, 2005), and concentrate on analysis of thoughts, ideas, and concepts (Clark & Holt, 2001). Philosophies and theories of nursing have been used in nursing curricula to clarify what nursing is, what should be studied, and how nursing differs from other disciplines (Uys and Smit, 1994). Philosophies of nursing include basic premises about the nature and goals of nursing, rights and obligations for health, and the role of nurses in society and in health care systems. Accordingly, mega-theories such as Rogers' life processes and Orem's self-care have been used as theoretical and philosophical bases of curricula. In contrast to these ideas, Bevis (2000) suggested that a philosophy may not be necessary, and that curriculum developers could substitute assumptions instead.

Although a philosophy for nursing education continues to be supported by curriculum developers, there are some difficulties in how it is used in curricula. For example, statements might not be acceptable to all stakeholders, be incongruent with the focus of the curriculum, be idealistic rather than real, be static, and too general (Torres & Stanton, 1982). As well, philosophy statements may lack meaning and not be shared with students, particularly if these statements are viewed merely as a professional or discipline requirement (Kintgen-Andrews, 1988). To ensure that the philosophy reflects faculty beliefs and values, and is relevant to social, cultural, professional, and consumer needs, it should be reviewed and updated periodically (Rentschler & Spegman, 1996).

Traditional Curriculum Philosophies

Although classical philosophies date back some 2500 years to Greek scholars of the 6th century BCE, differences in the philosophical bases of various disciplines began only in the last two centuries (Uys & Smit, 1994). For example, it was not until late into the 19th century that the first well-rounded philosophy about nursing education was developed by Florence Nightingale (Csokasy, 2005). In spite of the development of philosophies specific to disciplines, traditional schools of philosophy (i.e., *idealism* and *realism*) emanating from early Greek philosophers, still affect nursing education today.

Idealism According to this philosophy, truth is universal, values are unchanging, and individuals desire to live in a perfect world of high ideals, beauty, and art. The curriculum is built on humanism, liberal arts education, and promotion of intellectual growth. Teachers serve as role models for students, who are encouraged to think and expand their minds by applying knowledge to life.

Realism The main tenet of realism is that natural laws compose the world and regulate all of nature. Curriculum, therefore, is structured to present these universal laws. The curriculum is organized around content. Teachers provide information sequentially, in an efficient, simple-to-complex manner. According to this philosophy, students are motivated to learn through positive reinforcement, and rewarded for learning basic skills and responding to new experiences with scientific objectivity and analysis.

Learning Theories as Curriculum Philosophies

One or more learning theories could be used as the philosophical base and learning orientation of the nursing curriculum. The theory selected should reflect stakeholder views about learning, teaching, student characteristics, and the educational environment.

An example of a learning theory used as a philosophical base for the curriculum is *behaviorism*. This learning theory is grounded in *positivism*, the predominant form of scientific reasoning from the latter 19th century to the mid-20th century. With behaviorism, which was the foundation of nursing curricula for much of the 20th century, preeminence is given to behavioral objectives, positive reinforcement, and reward. Curricula are characterized by presentation of real facts and observable phenomena. The responsibility for organizing knowledge lies with the teacher. Students are largely passive learners and there is limited facilitation of critical analysis, thinking, reasoning, or creativity. Emphases are on students' ability to learn content and transfer formal propositional knowledge into clinical practice, which is generally supervised. Personal development is secondary (Yorks & Sharoff, 2001).

Other learning theories can be conceived as all or part of a philosophical base for a nursing curriculum. Vandeveer and Norton (2005) proposed that cognitive theories, cognitive development, multiple intelligences, some educational frameworks, and interpretive pedagogies could be used as frameworks for curriculum philosophy.

Current Nursing Curriculum Philosophies

The following philosophies, albeit merely highlighted, evidence some differences, but also commonalities. As can be detected, there is a blending of philosophy and learning theory, as well as an intermingling of beliefs, values, and teaching and learning applications.

Apprenticeship Hilton (2001) proposes an *apprenticeship* philosophy based on the epistemology of Michael Polanyi, the Hungarian scientist and philosopher. Polanyi (as cited in Hilton) believes that skills and ways of thinking are learned from experts with intuitive knowledge, and by example from authority figures (masters), in an apprenticeship arrangement. This is combined with holistic learning which takes place by seeing, doing, touching, experiencing, and by acquiring motor skills first, then building upon them. Using this approach, nursing students would begin with foundation courses (nursing fundamentals), and once they demonstrate mastery of laboratory skills and theoretical knowledge, would proceed with more difficult material in classrooms, laboratories, and clinical situations. Hilton recommends pairing students as apprentices with experienced nurses throughout the nursing curriculum, in accordance with Polanyi's views.

Similarly, *cognitive apprenticeship* is a teaching-learning experience in which students participate with experts in a community of practice, to learn expert knowledge, physical skills, procedures, thinking processes, and the culture of the field. Students observe, participate, and discover expert practice through teaching strategies such as modeling, coaching, scaffolding (hints, directions, reminders, physical assistance), and learning strategies such as articulation, reflection, and exploration (Taylor & Care, 1999).

Collaborative Inquiry Collaborative inquiry is a systemic process derived from whole-person epistemology. Students use experiences to generate new knowledge by action and reflection. Teachers and students share power and responsibility for decision-making. Critical subjectivity in the mutual pursuit of new meaning is practiced, and explicit activity procedures are followed. It draws on all four ways of knowing (empirical, ethical, personal, esthetic) (Carper, 1978), and legitimizes transformative and holistic learning early in the careers of nursing students.

Constructivism According to this view, knowledge is seen as constructed and all learning as connected. Reality is perceived as invented. The underlying knowledge base and questions arising from it are examined. Meanings resulting from the process of constructing knowledge could vary, depending on the context in which questions are asked and the frame of reference of the questioner (Belenky, Clinchy, Goldberger, & Tarule, cited in Walton, 1996).

Post-positivism Recent post-positivism perspectives also center on knowledge and meaning as opposed to prediction and control. Learning and meaning are seen to occur in the context and experience of the evolving co-constructed process between and among nurses, clients, teachers, and students (Walton, 1996). Learning and meaning-making involve connecting the view of others to one's own knowledge, and building a new co-constructed understanding of the shared experience (Surrey, as cited in Walton, 1996).

Critical Social Theory Critical social theory is concerned with justice, equality, and freedom. It maintains that knowledge as truth is socially constructed, and facts are relevant only in the lived experiences of persons (Duchscher, 2000). The premise is that all meanings and truths are interpreted in the context of social history (Henderson, 1995). Understanding patterns of human behavior involves knowledge of existing social structures and the communication processes that define them. Critical social theory enables students and faculty to share a revisioning and reconstruction of former potentially oppressive and coercive ideologies. Nurse educators encourage, listen, express, problem-pose, and philosophize to foster a critical approach to learning. Learners are assisted to take the role of others and develop empathy, confidence, and competence in human relations. These abilities develop through critical self-reflection, self-transformation, discussion, and dialogue (Duchscher).

Epistemology An epistemological philosophy emphasizes the relationship between persons and knowledge. Since much significant learning occurs apart from formal educational experiences, informal and incidental learning from lived experiences account for most learning. Students shape learning through established ways of knowing, such as experience, intuition, intellect, and practice (Heron, 1992).

Feminism   Feminism is an ideology originally premised on values and beliefs about women and relationships of gender. Feminist pedagogy serves as a means for educational development and social change to meet educational needs of women. More broadly interpreted, feminism values persons regardless of gender, with the goal of ending previous dehumanizing polarizations. It provides a framework that promotes development of intellectual growth and activism, and incorporates professional nursing values such as self-awareness, independence, empowerment, caring, and nursing's patterns of knowing. Students question, reflect, and challenge values and assumptions of nursing practice. Together with teachers, they co-construct meaning from life experiences. Students are empowered and test ideas through critical thinking, analysis, synthesis, and self-evaluation.

Humanism   A philosophy of humanism is concerned with rights, autonomy, and dignity of human beings. In a *humanistic-existentialist* curriculum, the focus is on personal meaning in human existence (Csokasy, 2005). Teachers question the need for outcome assessment, and rely instead on critical thinking, application of knowledge, and students' interpretation of the learning experience. The role of the teacher is to motivate and encourage experiential learning and facilitate students to establish and attain their own goals.

Interpretive Inquiry and Relational Humanistic Nursing   Interpretive inquiry and relational humanistic nursing (relational practice) is a process of intense reflection on events and experiences in which nursing students are part of a relational process of interpreting those events and experiences (Doanne, 2002). Students are not hampered by the ideas and content of a situation, the interpretation of the content, and what is to be done. Rather, the content becomes whatever arises through the inquiry process. Students authentically connect with their "self in relation" by inquiring into and interpreting their relational experiences and practices, and move beyond the self through reflection, dialogue, and reenactment.

Life Skills   Life skills philosophy is based on the premise that knowledge and facts can be quickly outdated, so students should learn and practice basic skills they will need for a lifetime. These basic skills support acquisition and integration of new knowledge as it is generated, enabling learners to take on new information and adapt to future change. Teaching methods are compatible with producing the workforce of the future, and incorporate a variety of participative learning strategies (Freeman, Voignier, & Scott, 2002).

Phenomenology   Phenomenology is an orientation and research method that focuses on lived experience and personal meaning. It emphasizes that people are always situated within a context, that there are multiple realities, and that people's perception of their experiences are valid. In nursing education, consideration is given to the experience of the individual (student, client, teacher), and learning experiences and the curriculum are framed in relation to these experiences.

Pragmatism   Central to pragmatism is the testing of ideas, a combination of idealism and realism. Pragmatism in education is based on *progressive* and *reconstructive* theories, whereby students are actively engaged in learning and exploring, in laboratory work, simulations, field trips, and social and community activities. Accountability is stressed, as learners develop new ideas, design the evaluation process, and undergo examinations. Learners are encouraged to take in new information, interpret and apply it to previous learning and current client experiences (Csokasy, 2002). Learning outcomes are assessed through observation of learners interacting with clients.

The preceding is merely an overview, since it is beyond the scope of this book to provide a comprehensive description of philosophies. The philosophies, singly or in combination, give rise to implications for nursing education. These are summarized in Table 7.1.

Philosophical Approaches

It is our view that the curriculum should be built on a philosophical base which is then embodied throughout the curriculum. Since most if not all nursing education curricula are based on ideas drawn from several philosophies, the term *philosophical approach(es)* seems more fitting than *philosophy*. This conceptualization implies a liberal interpretation of *philosophy* and can encompass eclecticism, pluralism, assumptions, beliefs, and values. Latitude and diversity in thoughts, views, values, assumptions, principles, and beliefs are thus possible. There must, however, be logical consistency in the espoused philosophical approaches. As well, they must be congruent with the values of faculty and the educational institution. Philosophical approaches can be expressed through philosophical or value statements, or through assumptions.

Developing Philosophical Approaches

The philosophical approaches subcommittee can begin by conducting a literature search and reviewing the philosophical statements of other schools of nursing. An early decision is whether to use a formal philosophy (or more than one), philosophical approaches, value statements, or assumptions.

The subcommittee should strive to understand the beliefs and values of colleagues, since all faculty implement the curriculum. A template could be given to faculty and other stakeholders, with a request that they write their beliefs about matters such as teaching and learning, the nature and purpose of student-faculty and nurse-client relationships, and so forth. Common ideas within the responses could be the basis of the curriculum's philosophical approaches. Another strategy could be to summarize the main precepts of several philosophies and request that stakeholders indicate those that best fit their ideas about nursing education. A third activity might be to delineate the teaching and learning implications of several philosophical approaches, and seek information about stakeholders' preferences.

TABLE 7.1   IMPLICATIONS OF PHILOSOPHICAL APPROACHES FOR NURSING EDUCATION

Philosophical Approaches	Key Ideas for Curriculum	Implications for Learners
Apprenticeship; Cognitive apprenticeship	Master-apprentice relationship; learning by example and from intuition of experts	Learn by example from experienced clinicians early in the curriculum and throughout the curriculum
Behaviorism/positivism	Positive reinforcement and reward; simple to complex curriculum; scientific objectivity; achievement of behavioral objectives	Motivated to learn by positive reinforcement and reward; learn content and transfer knowledge to clinical experience; able to practice as graduates if prescribed curriculum objectives and standards are met
Collaborative inquiry	Generation of new knowledge from reflection, shared power, active learning, and decision-making; four ways of knowing	Use of all four ways of knowing; use experiences to generate new knowledge
Critical social theory	Meanings and truth are interpreted in context of history; critical self-reflection develops capacity to examine experience in different ways; involves autonomy, social responsibility, emancipation, empowerment, and understanding	Share in revisioning and reconstructing formerly oppressive or coercive ideologies and practices
Constructivism; Post-positivism	Meaning and knowledge are constructed; learning is connected; new understandings occur between and among students, teachers, and clients	Construct knowledge by taking own and others' views to build new knowledge and a co-constructed understanding; learning and meaning-making arise from connecting others' views to own knowledge
Epistemology	Relationship between learner and knowledge; informal, incidental, lived experience learning	Comprehend that a relationship exists between self and knowledge, and informal, incidental, and lived experiences form most of learning

Feminism	Lived experiences; creative and critical thinking; empowerment	Empowered to question, reflect, challenge values and assumptions of nursing practice; incorporate life experience in learning
Humanism-existentialism	Critical thinking; application of knowledge; "being" in nursing; experiential learning	Motivated towards experiential learning; establishing and meeting own goals
Interpretive inquiry and relational humanism	Reflection on events, experiences, relations with others; process of interpreting content, content stems from inquiry process	Apply critical thinking and knowledge to interpret experiences; unhampered by ideas and content; reflect intensively on experiences and practices
Life skills	New knowledge acquisition and adaptation to future change; active learning; variety of participative learning strategies; skills and culture of nursing learned from experts in the field	Concern about large amount to learn; acquire information and skills to practice in the future
Phenomenology	Lived experiences; personal meaning and multiple realities	Derive personal meaning and learning from own lived experiences and those of others
Pragmatism	Observation and interpretation of face-to-face client interaction; active engagement in learning; self-evaluation; accountability; interpretation of new information applied to previous learning	Actively engage in learning; observe and assess self while interacting with others

Once information is obtained from stakeholders, philosophical approaches for the curriculum can be drafted and distributed with a request for feedback. Considerable discussion and several drafts are generally required before agreement is reached about the philosophical approaches.

The following questions could be considered when developing the philosophical approaches for the nursing curriculum:

- How can we become more knowledgeable about philosophical approaches in general education and nursing education?
- Should a single, pluralistic, or eclectic approach; value statements; or assumptions be used for the curriculum? What are the advantages and disadvantages of each?
- How can stakeholders' views be determined in a reasonable time period?
- Which philosophical approaches seem most consistent with the beliefs and values of stakeholders and the educational institution?
- What are the curriculum implications of the philosophical approaches we prefer?

The importance of consensus among the Total Faculty Group about the philosophical approaches cannot be over-emphasized. The philosophical approaches are the basis of the entire curriculum. There must be agreement and a common understanding about philosophical approaches when curriculum directions and outcomes are defined, and before subsequent curriculum work is undertaken. Time spent on reaching a shared understanding and agreement is time well spent. Once this is achieved, the philosophical approaches subcommittee can attend to perfecting the written statements.

Curriculum Goals

Curriculum goals are a public statement of the characteristics and competencies of graduates. The goals incorporate the philosophical approaches, curriculum directions, and curriculum outcomes. They are statements about the abilities and attitudes to be achieved by students, as well as the context in which these will be expressed. The term *goals* is used in this book to refer to the broad statements that reflect the substance of the nursing curriculum and describe the destination to be reached by graduating students. Various schools of nursing may refer to *terminal objectives, outcomes,* or *ends-in-view* to convey the same idea.

Purpose of Curriculum Goals for Various Audiences

The goals, which appear in published descriptions of the curriculum, have several audiences; each reads the goals for a different purpose. Curriculum builders, faculty members, current and prospective students, clinicians and potential employers, other members of the educational institution, representatives of accrediting organizations, provincial licensing bodies, and state boards of nursing, as well as members of professional nursing organizations, all have legitimate interest in curriculum goals.

Curriculum Developers This group uses the goals as a source of direction for all subsequent aspects of curriculum planning, implementation, and evaluation. This implies that the curriculum design, level and course goals, learning activities and assignments, and evaluation of learning all derive their focus and intent from the curriculum goals. Curriculum developers are obligated to create learning experiences that will allow motivated and capable students to achieve the curriculum goals.

Faculty Faculty designing individual courses turn to curriculum goals (from which more specific level and course goals emanate) as their reference point for all teaching and learning encounters and assessments of student learning. Goals are the standards for students to achieve and against which faculty assess the suitability of learning experiences.

Current Students Students enrolled in a school of nursing look to the curriculum goals as the target they should reach by graduation, and course goals as targets for smaller units of learning. To make goals meaningful to students, faculty should refer to them frequently, identifying how particular learning activities contribute to goal achievement. In this way, the goals have an educational value to students, and are not merely published statements that seem unrelated to courses. Additionally, frequent and explicit reference to curriculum goals helps students articulate their abilities and achievements.

Prospective Students Potential applicants can review the published goals to determine if the curriculum will match their view of nursing, personal expectations, and philosophical orientation. A curriculum that uses feminist approaches, for example, may be very attractive to some, and unappealing to others. Similarly, goals that reflect an emphasis on community health could attract those interested in working in non-institutional settings, while prospective students interested in critical care would be unlikely to apply. Published goals can help attract students whose interests are aligned with the curriculum purposes and processes.

Clinicians and Potential Employers These groups can use the published goal statements to understand, in general terms, what students are expected to accomplish and what abilities they will have at graduation. Reference to goals by faculty can be effective in helping clinicians appreciate why the nursing curriculum may not prepare students in the manner clinicians might prefer. Similarly, goals that include curriculum concepts such as critical thinking, reflective and collaborative practice, or leadership could assist employers to recognize the value graduates can bring to organizations, following a suitable period of orientation.

Other Members of the Educational Institution Faculty teaching support courses, chairs of institution-wide committees concerned with curricula and standards, and administrators, are interested in whether the nursing curriculum goals are congruent with the mission, goals, and values of the educational institution. If institution-wide outcomes have been delineated for programs, these should be apparent in the curriculum goals, although presented within the context of nursing. However, nursing curriculum goals might exceed those of the institution.

Representatives of Accrediting Organizations, State Boards of Nursing, and Provincial Licensing Bodies Representatives of organizations concerned with nursing education and nursing practice standards are also interested in the curriculum goals. They want to be assured that the goals match the expectations for the program level (practical nursing, associate degree, diploma, or baccalaureate). Additionally, curriculum goals, among other information, are evaluated when graduates seek licensure in jurisdictions other than where they were originally licensed.

Members of Professional Nursing Organizations These persons review nursing curriculum goals to keep abreast of educational expectations and abilities of new graduates. Changes in curriculum goals might form part of the rationale used to substantiate recommendations to legislators about nursing practice and health care policy.

Members of the Public Health care recipients generally read curriculum goals only when they encounter a problem in nursing practice. In those instances, if a complaint to a licensing body or a lawsuit is considered, members of the public and/or their legal representatives may want to determine the curriculum goals graduates should have achieved.

Formulating Curriculum Goals

As previously stated, curriculum goals are developed from the agreed-upon philosophical approaches and curriculum directions and outcomes, all of which should be evident in the goal statements. The curriculum goals must be congruent with the mission and goals of the school of nursing and educational institution. There could be considerable similarity in the curriculum goals of many schools of nursing because curriculum developers are guided by similar contextual influences, such as nursing practice or performance standards; codes of ethics; licensure and accreditation requirements; provincial, state, or national positions on higher education; and prevailing educational philosophies. Yet, as much as possible, the goals should give an indication of the uniqueness of each school's curriculum.

The language and format of the goal statements must be consistent with the philosophical approaches, and must reflect predominant curriculum directions and outcomes. When writing goals, curriculum developers need to be mindful not only of student outcomes, but also of the audiences for the goals, and should ensure that the terminology is understandable to those who are not current with the language of nursing education. The goal statements should be comprehensive, yet concrete enough to be meaningful, and broad enough to allow for ongoing curriculum refinement.

Synthetic thinking, artful writing, and ongoing discussion among faculty are required for goal statements that reflect the intent of the curriculum. The subcommittee preparing the goals should be immersed in the philosophical approaches, curriculum directions and curriculum outcomes, nursing education and practice standards, and other relevant information assembled as part of the contextual data. Goal statements from other schools can also provide useful ideas.

When developing goal statements for the nursing curriculum, the goals subcommittee might consider the following:

- What format is compatible with the philosophical approaches: goals, terminal objectives, outcomes, ends-in-view?
- What are the most relevant nursing education and practice standards that must be evident (or exceeded) in the goals?
- How can graduates' abilities, and the context in which abilities will be evident, be meaningfully described?
- How can we ensure that the goals are appropriate for the program level and grounded in the philosophical approaches, curriculum outcomes, and curriculum directions?
- How can we expeditiously obtain feedback from stakeholders?

Formulating goals can be laborious and controversial. Because the goals encapsulate graduates' abilities, the use of unambiguous language is essential. Faculty members are rightfully concerned about accuracy, reasonableness, and comprehensiveness in the goal statements and, therefore, discussion about both the substance and phraseology can be expected before approval is achieved. Sample goals, based on humanistic-educative approaches, for a baccalaureate curriculum are presented in Table 7.2.

Faculty Development

Faculty development can focus on the purpose of philosophical approaches in the curriculum. Values and beliefs about nursing, education, persons, and so forth could be discussed. Examples of standard philosophies could be circulated to help those in attendance see what others have developed. Beginning belief and value statements could be drafted, and the purpose and formulation of goals could be addressed. Some practice with writing goals would be valuable, particularly if the format of the statements is changing from the existing one. Members experienced in curriculum development can facilitate these sessions.

Chapter Summary

The philosophical approaches of the nursing curriculum reflect the beliefs, values, and convictions of faculty. These approaches should be evident throughout the entire curriculum. The curriculum goals state the characteristics and abilities of graduates. Together, the philo-

---

TABLE 7.2   SAMPLE BACCALAUREATE CURRICULUM GOALS, BASED ON HUMANISTIC-EDUCATIVE APPROACHES

Using a humanistic-educative perspective, graduates will:

- practice evidence-based, ethical, competent nursing, incorporating health promotion perspectives and respect for the diversity and culture of individuals, families, and communities
- demonstrate leadership in planning, providing, managing, and evaluating care in institutional and community settings
- establish productive collegial relationships that support collaborative decision-making in planning care and resolving clinical problems
- promote justifiable positions to advance professional nursing practice and health care policies that are responsive to societal needs
- identify researchable problems and critique research relevant to nursing care and health care delivery

---

sophical approaches and goals form the basis of the nursing curriculum, and must be congruent with those of the educational institution.

In this chapter, the definition and purposes of a curriculum philosophy are presented. Some traditional and current curriculum philosophies are briefly described. The authors' view of philosophical approaches and how to develop these approaches for the curriculum are suggested. Similarly, the definition, purposes, and formulation of curriculum goals are described. Faculty development activities are suggested.

Synthesis Activities

As in other chapters, two cases are presented for review and discussion. The first case is critiqued; the second is for analysis. Following the cases, questions are offered about developing curriculum philosophies and goals, to guide curriculum development in individual settings.

Sanderson University

Sanderson University School of Nursing has been offering a 4-year baccalaureate nursing curriculum based on a single positivist philosophical approach. The related goals are that graduates will practice safe and competent nursing with multicultural groups, interact effectively with members of the health care team, participate in research activities, and advance nursing practice. Success rates over the past ten years on the NCLEX have ranged between 80–85%, demonstrating that graduates have met standards set by the school and licensure bodies.

The 16 faculty members, seven of whom were appointed within the last two years, have been lobbying for a change in the philosophical approaches and goals. With the cooperation of the Director of the School, they have proposed that either a pluralistic or eclectic philosophical approach be formulated to more clearly reflect their current beliefs and values about nursing, teaching and learning, and to incorporate changes inherent in health care and society.

After several months of discussions in faculty and curriculum committee meetings, all members have agreed to base the curriculum on more current approaches, and to express these in philosophical assumptions. The fundamental concepts of *person, health, nursing, nurse, nursing education,* and *learning* are to be retained as the framework for the philosophical approaches. A first draft of the philosophical assumptions based on these concepts has been distributed. The members have also affirmed that the goals should be broadly stated, incorporating the philosophical approaches, curriculum directions, and curriculum outcomes.

Critique The faculty have persisted in bringing about consensus to change the curriculum's philosophical approaches and goals. Several months of deliberation have resulted in a draft of the philosophical assumptions. Their perseverance, together with the cooperation of the Director of the School, is commendable. They have reached unanimity about the philosophical approaches, a significant milestone in curriculum development. There is much work yet to be done.

It would have been advisable, however, for the faculty and curriculum committee to come to agreement about which contemporary approach(es) to use before preparing a draft. A review of contemporary philosophies and philosophical assumptions, therefore, would be in order. The curriculum committee leader or a consultant might assist in these discussions. It would also be worthwhile to take another look at the mission of the institution, examine contextual factors that would have a bearing on the revised philosophy and curriculum goals, and consider the audience for whom the goals would be relevant. Subcommittees could be appointed, one to continue the work of developing the philosophical assumptions, and another to formulate the curriculum goals.

Michaelson County Community College Case

Michaelson County Community College is one of two post-secondary institutions located in a small city with a largely working-class population of 39,000. One 150-bed general hospital, a 98-bed residential care facility, and two health clinics provide services to the community. The College offers one- and two-year certificate and associate-degree (AD) programs during day, evening, and weekend hours. Approximately 6400 full- and part-time students are enrolled in technology and health-related programs.

The associate-degree nursing (ADN) program is open to students who qualify after completing a high school diploma. The curriculum was first approved in 1976, and has since graduated over 1600 nurses. A 78% success rate on first-time attempts at NCLEX in the early years has increased to 85%.

The ADN curriculum has undergone several changes in keeping with new approaches in nursing education and practice. Mildred Spenser, MSN, RN, present director of the program, has been meeting for several months with the nursing faculty and the curriculum committee to discuss changes to the curriculum. They have been reviewing environmental, socio-economic, cultural, professional, and institutional factors related to the college, community, and the ADN program. Current curriculum development activity is focused on the philosophical approaches and curriculum goals.

Guided by the curriculum coordinator, the committee (comprised of faculty, students, and agency representatives) has already determined that apprenticeship or cognitive apprenticeship philosophical approaches would be suitable. They have drafted an updated, all-encompassing goal, i.e., that graduates will provide safe, ethical, culturally-sensitive nursing practice, and will work with other health care providers in the care of individuals, families, and communities. The intent now is to articulate more specifically the knowledge and competencies inherent in this goal. A schedule of future meetings has been posted.

Questions for Consideration and Analysis of Michaelson County Community College Case

1. What philosophical assumptions or statements can be derived from the apprenticeship or cognitive apprenticeship approaches?
2. How will these assumptions or statements guide the curriculum?
3. What effect will the philosophical assumptions have on the curriculum goals?
4. What must the curriculum committee do in order to consolidate the curriculum goals?
5. Consider the advantages and disadvantages of:
   - deriving knowledge and competencies from broad curriculum goals
   - deriving goals from philosophical approaches and curriculum directions and outcomes.
6. Formulate:
   - a description of the apprenticeship or cognitive apprenticeship philosophical approaches for the ADN curriculum
   - ADN curriculum goals based on apprenticeship or cognitive apprenticeship philosophical approaches

Curriculum Development Activities for Consideration in Your Setting

The questions below are intended to stimulate thinking about developing philosophical approaches and formulating curriculum goals in your setting.

1. What influence will the contextual factors have on the envisioned philosophical approaches and curriculum goals?
2. Who should be involved in the development of the philosophical approaches and curriculum goals?
3. How should the development of philosophical approaches and goals for the curriculum proceed?
4. Which philosophical approaches, traditional or contemporary, would be consistent with our ideas, beliefs, convictions, and values?
5. What philosophy or philosophical approaches would be most appropriate for the nursing curriculum as we envision it?
6. If faculty members ascribe to more than one philosophical approach, would an eclectic or a pluralistic approach more clearly express our views?
7. How can we assure that our philosophical approaches are congruent with those of the educational institution?
8. How can we articulate our philosophical approaches and curriculum goals?
9. What do we need to keep in mind when writing the curriculum goals?
10. How can we assure that the curriculum goals reflect the philosophical approaches and curriculum directions and outcomes?
11. What resources will be required to complete the philosophical approaches and curriculum goals?
12. What is a reasonable time period for completion of these curriculum elements?
13. What faculty development activities could help us develop the philosophical approaches and curriculum goals?

References

Bevis, E.O. (1986). *Curriculum building in nursing. A process.* (3rd ed.). St. Louis: C.V. Mosby Co.
Bevis, E.O. (2000). Illuminating the issues. In E.O. Bevis & J. Watson (Eds.), *Toward a caring curriculum. A new pedagogy for nursing.* (pp. 13–35). Boston: Jones and Bartlett Publishers.

Carper, B.A. (1978). Fundamental patterns of knowing in nursing. *Advances in Nursing Science, 1,* 13–23.

Clark, D., & Holt, J. (2001). Philosophy: A key to open the door to critical thinking. *Nurse Education Today, 21,* 71–78.

Clayton, G.M. (1989). Curriculum revolution: Defining the concepts. *Journal of Professional Nursing, 5*(1), 6, 55.

Csokasy, J. (2002). A congruent curriculum philosophical integrity from philosophy to outcomes. *Journal of Nursing Education, 41*(1), 32–33.

Csokasy, J. (2005). Philosophical foundations of the curriculum. In D. Billings & J. Halstead (Eds.), *Teaching in nursing: A guide for faculty.* (2nd ed.). (pp. 125–143). St. Louis: Elsevier Saunders.

Dillard, N., Sitkberg, L., & Laidig, J. (2005). Curriculum development. An overview. In D.M. Billings & J. Halstead (Eds.), *Teaching in nursing. A guide for faculty.* (2nd ed.). (pp. 89–107). St. Louis: Elsevier Saunders.

Duchscher, J.E.B. (2000). Bending a habit: Critical social theory as a framework for humanistic nursing education. *Nurse Education Today, 20,* 453–462.

Doanne, G.A.H. (2002). Beyond behavioral skills to human-involved processes. Relational nursing practice and interpretive pedagogy. *Journal of Nursing Education , 41*(8), 400–404.

Freeman, L.H., Voignier, R.R., & Scott, D.L. (2002). New curriculum for a new century: Beyond repackaging. *Journal of Nursing Education, 41*(1), 36–40.

Gates, R. (1990). From educational philosophy to educational practice: Fidelity and the curriculum in context. *Nurse Education Today, 10,* 420–427.

Haynes, L., Boese, T., & Butcher, H. (2004). *Nursing in contemporary society. Issues, trends, and transition to practice.* Upper Saddle River, NJ: Pearson Prentice Hall.

Henderson, D.J. (1995). Consciousness-raising in participatory research: Method and methodology for emancipatory inquiry. *Advances in Nursing Science, 17,* 58–69.

Heron, J. (1992). *Feeling and personhood. Psychology in another key.* Newbury Park, CA: Sage.

Hilton, J.J. (2001). Polanyi's philosophy. A new look at a theoretical framework. *Nurse Educator, 27,* 249–250.

Kintgen-Andrews, J. (1988). Philosophy statements: Challenging beliefs and values. *Nursing and Health Care, 9,* 436–438.

Lawrence, S.A., & Lawrence, R.M. (1983). Curriculum development: Philosophy, objectives, and conceptual framework. *Nursing Outlook, 3,* 160–163.

Marriner-Tomey, A. (1988). *Guide to nursing management.* (3rd Ed.) St. Louis: C.V. Mosby.

Petress, K. (2003). An educational philosophy guides the pedagogical process. *College Student Journal, 37*(1), 128–135.

Rentschler, D.D., & Spegman, A.M. (1996). Curriculum revolution. Realities of change. *Journal of Nursing Education, 35*(9), 389–393.

Taylor, K.L., & Care, D.W. (1999). Nursing education as cognitive apprenticeship. *Nurse Educator, 24*(4), 31–36.

Torres, G., & Stanton, M. (1982). *Curriculum process in nursing.* Englewood Cliffs, N.J.: Prentice-Hall.

Tyler, R.W. (1949). *Basic principles of curriculum and instruction.* Chicago: University of Chicago Press.

Uys, L.R., & Smit, J.H. (1994). Writing a philosophy of nursing. *Journal of Advanced Nursing, 20,* 239–244.

Vandeveer, M., & Norton, B. (2005). From teaching to learning. Theoretical foundations. In D. Billings & J. Halstead (Eds.), *Teaching in nursing: A guide for faculty.* (2nd ed.). (pp. 231–281). St. Louis: Elsevier Saunders.

Walton, J.C. (1996). The changing environment. New challenges for nursing education. *Journal of Nursing Education, 35*(9), 400–405.

White, B., & Brockett, R. (1987). Putting philosophy into practice. *Journal of Extension, 25*(2), available from *www.joe.org.*

Wiles, J., & Bondi, J. (2002). *Curriculum development. A guide to practice.* (5th ed.) Upper Saddle Printer, New Jersey: Merrill.

Yorks, L., & Sharoff, L. (2001). An extended epistemology for fostering transformative learning in holistic nursing education. *Holistic Nursing Practice, 16*(1), 21–29.

Yura, H. (1974). Curriculum development process. In *Faculty curriculum development. Part 1: The process of curriculum development.* New York: National League for Nursing.

CHAPTER 8

Curriculum Design

Chapter Overview

In this chapter, information about curriculum design is presented first. Included are terminology, descriptions about program delivery, program models, organizing strategies for curriculum design, and patterns for course sequencing. These provide background to the section on the *process* of curriculum design, in which attention is given to parameters of the design, facilitating the process, and selecting delivery approaches, a program model, an organizing strategy, and course sequencing. Identifying courses is addressed. This is followed by consideration of program policies and human and financial implications. Although presented in a linear fashion, curriculum design does not occur through a prescribed sequence, but rather through iterative discussion, generation of design ideas, and critique. Following a brief discussion of faculty development related to curriculum design and a chapter summary, two cases are presented. The first case is critiqued; the second is for analysis. Questions to determine curriculum design activities in individual settings conclude the chapter.

Chapter Goals

- Understand the process of curriculum design
- Identify factors important in curriculum design decisions
- Appreciate variations in curriculum design

- Consider human and financial implications of curriculum design
- Reflect on faculty development activities pertinent to curriculum design

Curriculum Design

The term, *curriculum design*, when used as a noun, refers to the configuration of the program of studies. It is frequently understood to be the listing of courses that appears in the institutional calendar. However, the design encompasses the courses, their sequencing, the relationships between and among courses, and associated curriculum policies.

The *process of designing the curriculum*, or the *curriculum design process*, refers to the discussions and decision-making that lead to the configuration of the program of studies. This process can feel like the heart of curriculum development. The design makes tangible the completed work and the future curriculum. Curriculum developers can feel a strong sense of accomplishment and satisfaction when they are able to say, "This is our curriculum."

As the design process begins, it is valuable to clarify expectations of this aspect of curriculum development, since members of the development team may have different outlooks about design and what it entails. As in all of curriculum development, similarities should be capitalized upon, previous decisions recalled, and differences negotiated. It is worthwhile to review the curriculum work done to date in order to rekindle common perspectives.

The design must be congruent with the philosophical approaches chosen for the curriculum and provide opportunities for students to achieve curriculum goals. This should be uppermost in all deliberations about design. Sequencing, continuity, integration of concepts, responsiveness to contextual factors, and attention to students' multiple ways of knowing are other design considerations to be kept in mind. Concurrent with the curriculum design process is the creation of a plan for evaluation, an important and often overlooked aspect of curriculum development (see Chapter 10 for a discussion of evaluation planning).

It may be helpful to clarify some of the terminology used when undertaking the design phase of curriculum development. Terms such as *design, structure*, and *model* are often used interchangeably in the nursing education literature. To add to the confusion, descriptors such as *block, integrated, 2 + 2*, or *collaborative* have been referred to as designs, programs, structures, models, or patterns. To provide conceptual clarity, the following interpretations are used in this book and are more fully described in the following sections.

A program can be described according to its: *type*, (educational level, i.e., doctoral, masters, baccalaureate, associate degree, diploma, or practical nurse); *structure* (arrangement as to program length and semester or quarter divisions); *delivery* (means by which faculty offer the curriculum to students); and *model* (overall organization of the curriculum which typically describes the arrangement of nursing and support courses, e.g., articulated or upper division nursing program). These design elements affect the configuration of courses.

Program Type and Structure

The *program type*, or educational level, has a significant influence on the curriculum design, since the number of courses and the nature of learning experiences will be guided by the goals relevant to differing educational levels. The program type should be foremost in the minds of curriculum designers. It should be evident in the curriculum goals, which should be internalized by curriculum planners. Design proposals must be congruent with curriculum goals.

Program structure refers to the duration of the program and the arrangement of divisions within the academic year. The duration is usually a function of program type, although alternative program lengths can be considered, such as an accelerated baccalaureate program which can be 12 to 18 months in length (Shiber, 2003). Once established, the program length is a boundary within which the curriculum must be designed. The division of the academic year into quarters, semesters, or terms is established by the educational institution. These divisions are the temporal units in which semester and course goals must be achievable.

Program Delivery

Program delivery, another design element, refers to the means by which faculty offer the curriculum to students. Traditionally, this has been through provision of courses at the educational institution that awards the academic credential. Now, however, programs are extended through distance delivery and partnerships.

Traditional Delivery

The traditional approach for delivering nursing curricula has been face-to-face instruction, in which the teacher and students are physically present in the same classroom or clinical learning environment, at the same time, for a designated time period. This time- and place-dependent approach has evolved to include more flexible delivery. For example, faculty can travel to distant locations to offer classes to students unable to attend the educational institution, or clinical placements can be negotiated in students' home communities. Availability of faculty resources and costs associated with time and travel are some issues related to flexible, traditional delivery.

Distance Delivery

Distance education is a broad term that suggests there is a geographic distance separating students (individually or collectively) from the instructor and program of interest. "Distance education, distance teaching, distance learning, open learning, distributed learning, asynchronous learning, telelearning, and flexible learning are some of the terms used to describe an educational process in which the teacher and students are physically separated" (Picciano, 2001, p. 4).

Distance education provides access for students who prefer the flexible approaches that can accommodate their learning styles and multiple life roles. A paced course, typical in undergraduate and degree completion programs, is completed in a specified time period. Alternatively, if the course is not paced, students have more flexibility in timing. Many variations are possible in the execution of distance courses, although they normally include the use of technology to connect students with faculty and each other. Course materials can be print-based, computer-based, video- and audio-taped, or a combination of these. The following are some examples of the commonly-used distance delivery modes.

Correspondence Courses   Correspondence courses are place-independent. Course materials and assignments are mailed to students, who then return assignments to the course instructor for grading. This approach has been popular for many years and although students normally can have regular contact with faculty by mail, phone, fax, or email, they lack the benefit of dialogue and ongoing interaction with faculty and other students.

Broadcast Television   Through satellite or local television networks, broadcast television provides synchronous (same time) delivery to students in different locations. Transmission of information flows primarily in one direction, from instructor to students. Although normally in their own homes, students could be at designated sites with others taking the same course. They can communicate with the instructor by mail, phone, fax, or email. If together, students have the added benefit of interaction, perhaps with the help of a tutor.

Video Conferencing   This delivery mode promotes two-way interaction between and among instructor and students. This method is time- and place-dependent, but can be delivered to multiple points simultaneously. As well, participants can dialogue with each other, depending on the course design.

Tele-Conferencing   Also referred to as audio conferencing, tele-conferencing is another synchronous delivery method that can be used to engage students in interaction. Place independence is possible, however, the technology is time-dependent because communication is through a telephone line. Group teleconferences require access to technology at designated locations.

Computer Conferencing   Computer conferencing is an electronic delivery method that connects students with the instructor in a shared learning space using computer technology. It can be synchronous (real-time) or asynchronous (delayed-time). With personal computers, participants connect to a host computer that stores all messages constructed during a discussion. These can be accessed, read, downloaded, reviewed, and reflected upon at any time by course participants. This many-to-many approach to learning promotes the development of multiple perspectives and shared understandings among students and is used in all levels of academia (Andrusyszyn, 1998; Harasim, Hiltz, Teles, & Turoff, 1995). In this medium, participants experience a sense of equality (Burge & Roberts, 1993), since each participant has an equal voice in knowledge construction.

Hybrid Approaches Two or more delivery approaches are also possible in a curriculum or within individual courses. For example, some portions of a course could employ video conferencing, while others may require asynchronous computer conferencing. Course materials on CD-ROM, or available on the Internet with links to multiple websites, might be chosen to support course goals. As well, computer conferencing could be used as a complement to any other distance education method, or to classroom and clinical courses, when additional interaction among participants is desired.

Delivery Through Partnerships

Partnerships are formal arrangements that exist between and among institutions. In the nursing education literature, the terms *partnership, collaboration, collaborative partnership,* and *consortia* are often used without sufficient definition or differentiation. They do, however, refer to formal or informal affiliations or alliances developed by educational institutions with service agencies for student clinical experiences, or to arrangements that exist between and among educational institutions for the purpose of providing nursing education.

Partnerships among educational institutions are formed when more than one institution offers all or part of the same program. These agreements require a high level of trust and cooperation. In collaborative partnerships and consortia, in which there is a common curriculum, negotiations and a willingness to let go of treasured aspects of individual programs are necessary to achieve shared educational goals. Contractual arrangements typically specify the responsibilities of all parties in developing, approving, implementing, and evaluating the curriculum, including financial provisions. Additionally, details about the curriculum design can be specified.

The nature of the contractual arrangements can have a profound effect on curriculum design. Clauses about design (such as where, how, and which courses will be offered), as well as resource sharing and requirements about faculty credentials could be written to ensure curriculum quality. However, the more specific the curriculum detail in the signed agreements and the greater the number of institutions involved, the more difficult it can be to modify the curriculum as time passes. Curriculum revision or complete change will require approval from all partners, and possibly new contracts. Therefore, it may be wise to minimize references to specific design details when agreements are first developed.

Three principal forms of partnerships exist between and among educational institutions. They are fee-for-service, collaborative, and consortium partnerships.

Fee-for-Service Partnership This agreement is the least complex. One institution might purchase a course from a second institution. Elements of the contract could include the nature of the course, number of students, delivery mode(s), and the fee, which would be based on enrollment numbers. The provider is unlikely to participate in the purchaser's curriculum development. If the provider becomes unable to offer the course, the purchaser's curriculum might be compromised.

Collaborative Partnership A collaborative partnership denotes a higher degree of involvement between (or among) educational institutions. The collaborating partners share in curriculum development, implementation, and evaluation. Many different contractual arrangements are possible to achieve shared educational goals.

For example, in the Canadian province of Ontario, beginning January 2005, a nursing baccalaureate degree is the entry to practice requirement. To achieve this goal, the colleges of applied arts and technology (which have offered diploma, not degree, nursing programs) have joined with universities to offer four-year collaborative baccalaureate programs. Universities have one or more college partners, with each partnership having one curriculum. The universities confer the degree. The formal arrangements, in which nursing is offered in all four years, include:

- 2 years at a college for all students, followed by 2 years at the university
- enrollment in either the college or university for the first 2 years of the program, with all students enrolled at the university for the final two years
- simultaneous enrollment in both the college and university, with all students taking courses at both sites throughout the four years
- simultaneous delivery of the entire program at each of the university and college sites

The degree of autonomy within the partnership about admissions policies and procedures, flexibility within the agreed-upon curriculum, sharing of resources, and other matters varies from partnership to partnership.

Consortium A consortium is a co-operative grouping of many partners to achieve common goals. An example is the statewide consortium of nursing programs being created in Oregon to double the number of nursing graduates. This is "a voluntary coalition of associate degree (ADN) and public and private baccalaureate degree (BSN) programs" (Gubrud-Howe et al., 2003, p.166). In this consortium, a common curriculum is being planned, culminating in a BSN degree, although community college students will be able to receive an ADN degree and write National Council Licensure Examination (NCLEX) before completing the BSN at a university. The intent is to share faculty, laboratories, classrooms, and learning resources across nursing programs. Distance and web-based learning will give all students access to expert teachers and common learning experiences.

Program Models

The *program model* is the overall organization of the curriculum. This organization can vary according to arrangement and numbers of learning activities (nursing, non-nursing support and elective courses, clinical experiences) and program length, but all models are designed to meet the overall goals of the program. In essence, the model determines where learning activities can be placed in the program. The name given to the model may include a reference to the program length. It is important not to confuse *program model* with conceptual model or paradigm.

One example of a model is a *four-year baccalaureate program,* with an *exit* option to write licensure examinations after 3 years. In this model, courses deemed essential for RN practice must be included in the first 3 years. The fourth year includes courses necessary to meet institutional requirements for the nursing degree. In a four-year *generic,* or *basic* program, nursing and support courses are given throughout the entire program, whereas in an *upper division* program, nursing courses are offered after foundation courses in other disciplines. *Integrated* programs combine or blend concepts so that courses are connected in a meaningful way (Pennington, 1986). *Articulated* programs have a planned progression from a lower to a higher level of learning, for example, LPN to ADN, ADN to BSN or MSN. *External* degree models, for ADN or BSN study, are not centered on traditional patterns of institutional-based study. Rather, the focus is on the concept of providing credit on the basis of what one knows, not on how one has achieved it.

The program model is an important element of design. If a nursing program is being created in an institution where nursing did not formerly exist, then there is freedom to choose the program model. However, if there is a desire to change an existing model, considerable negotiation may be required, since there can be budgetary implications for the school of nursing and other departments.

Organizing Strategies for Nursing Curriculum Design

Nursing has always used an organizing strategy for curriculum design, beginning with Nightingale's statements about the environment. Since then, numerous organizing strategies have been developed. The one selected should provide optimal usefulness and consistency; be responsive to current and future social contexts; and be congruent with the philosophical approaches. Boland (2005) emphasizes that the organizing strategy "must reflect the domain of nursing practice, the phenomena of concern to nurses, and how nurses relate to others who are dealing with health concerns" (p.168). In relation to curriculum, one criterion of The National League for Nursing Accrediting Commission (NLNAC) (2003) is that, "curriculum developed by faculty flows from the nursing education unit philosophy/mission through an organizing framework into a logical progression of course outcomes and learning activities to achieve desired program objectives/outcomes" (p.15).

Traditional Organizing Strategies

Medical Model   In the medical model of organizing nursing curricula, popular for more than half of the 20th century, content was organized according to the following components: disease (teaching by body system), knowledge (learning by parts and adding on), terms or vocabulary (precise definitions), concept of nurse (whose function is incidental and who 'does things' to the patient and environment), and concept of patient (as a repository of disease). In this organizing strategy, courses are ordered in specific sequences. The content to be learned and how it is to be learned are identified. Nursing courses and nursing skills are delineated first, then the support courses, critical learning experiences, and evaluation methods to assess what students have learned.

The traditional hospital clinical area is the focus of learning, with a possible addition of a community experience. Advantages of this organizing strategy include availability of nursing textbooks written according to the medical model, fit with hospital organization, and match with popular perceptions of nursing. Nursing knowledge, however, may not be given prominence in the curriculum.

Simple-to-Complex   In a simple-to-complex organizing strategy, another traditional approach, knowledge is organized so that learning occurs sequentially. Students learn progressively more about a specific concept or process over time. For example, the curriculum might first address nursing care of individuals, then families, then aggregate groups. The advantage rests with the innate logic of incremental learning: students are expected to be responsive first to one person, then to a small group, and then to a community. However, this organization does not reflect the reality of nursing practice, since nurses typically respond to families along with individuals, to individuals within families and groups, and to both individuals and small groups within aggregates.

Stages of Illness   Health and its meaning are considered first when employing stages of illness as the organizing strategy. Acute-care nursing, and then rehabilitative and chronic-care nursing follow. Normal life processes such as pregnancy and aging do not fit easily into this approach, nor does health promotion of families and groups. Nonetheless, this strategy can encompass both institutional and community-based practice.

Contemporary Organizing Strategies

Nursing Conceptual Framework, Model, or Theory The curriculum can be organized according to one nursing conceptual framework, model, or theory, for example Orem's theory
of self-care, Peplau's theory of interpersonal relationships, Leininger's cultural care, or Watson's
human science, human care. These can be employed individually. Each conceptual framework,
model, or theory offers a somewhat different perspective of nursing with accompanying vocabulary. With this organizing strategy, the concepts and components of the selected theory or
practice framework are predominant in all courses and experiences. The nursing focus is foremost in the curriculum and directs students to view theory and practice with a specific perspective. However, a single nursing conceptual framework, model, or theory may not reflect
the views of all faculty and students, and the language and critical concepts may be too abstract
for students. As well, textbooks and other references may not be organized according to the
chosen perspective.

Multiple or *eclectic nursing conceptual (or theoretical) frameworks* can also be adopted.
Curriculum designers select concepts and definitions that best fit their values and beliefs about
nursing. Using several conceptual frameworks, models, or theories within the curriculum (pluralism), or combining parts of two or more theories (eclecticism) might be less constrain-
ing than relying on only one. This would combine what is best understood from several nursing
frameworks, models or theories. Adaptation of elements from multiple perspectives could
generate creative curriculum designs. Nevertheless, a multiple approach could jeopardize the
body of knowledge from one model, or take away from that which is uniquely nursing.
Distortion of original concepts, definitions, characteristics, and attributes of one or more of
the original models or theories might result.

Other Theories, Concepts, and Philosophies Theories, concepts, and philosophies, which
influence the development of the curriculum philosophical approaches, could also be the basis of the curriculum design. For example, views related to theories of knowledge development,
domains of practice, feminism, phenomenology, and existentialism, singly or in combination,
can be used to organize the curriculum.

Variables, Cornerstones, or General Skill Categories Other organizing strategies have been
advanced, such as *variables, cornerstones,* or *general skill categories.* Burden of illness, groups at
risk, health factors, and relevant nursing interventions (Arthur & Baumann, 1996) are possible organizing *variables.* As well, *cornerstones,* such as nursing knowledge, skills, values, meanings, and experiences (Bayliss-Webber, 2002) could become a curriculum framework. Further,
general skill categories and accompanying competencies could be part of an organizing strategy for curriculum design. Skills such as communication, internal locus of control, legisla-
tive/policy awareness, leadership/influence, crisis management strategies, and organization
(Bowen, Lyons, & Young, 2000) could be used. *Life skills* (communication, assessment, inter-

vention, evaluation, systems management, and professional behavior) (Freeman, Voignier, & Scott, 2002) might also become an organizing framework for the curriculum. Cognitive skills of professional practice (artful design, conceptualization, fluid inquiry, reflective conversation, and cognitive frame analysis) have formed a framework for RN to BSN education (Eckhardt, Matthias Anderson, Campbell, Clarke, & Pavlish, 2002).

Outcomes An *outcomes* approach, in part shaped by National League for Nursing 1993 reforms, is still another organizing strategy. These *outcomes*, which could form components of the design, would include critical thinking, collaborative skills, shared decision-making, social and epidemiological viewpoints, analyses and interventions at systems and aggregate levels, shifts from traditional to humanistic-educative models, changes in health care and in higher education, and outcome student assessments (Boland, 2005). Conceivably, Lindeman's (2000) recommendations for the year 2005, based on changes in higher education and nursing practice, might also be viewed as an *outcome* design. These outcomes include well-developed cognitive skills, personal and professional development, interdisciplinary team membership, and knowledge and skill development for safe practice.

If curriculum developers are concerned with *outcomes* or *end-stages*, this might suggest that the curriculum design proceed from this point first, and work towards the usual beginning phase. In this way, curriculum designers would initially identify the *outcomes* students should demonstrate, and accordingly shape the concepts embedded in the *outcomes* and competencies. For example, if health promotion, critical thinking, collaborative skills, and shared decision-making (and others identified above) are necessary outcomes, these concepts or competencies will form components of the curriculum. This end-to-beginning organization, with a starting point on desired *outcomes* or competencies, is not only different from the more traditional approaches, but may also be more practical. Curriculum developers would first identify essential qualities of graduates, then competencies or competency statements in each year of the program necessary to attain the *outcomes* (which also become the evaluation criteria), the antecedents or factors necessary for achieving the competencies, the learning experiences, teaching methods, learning resources, and assessment strategies (Boland, 1998; 2005).

Multi-, Inter-, and Trans-Disciplinary Models In these models, all health science professional programs share or collaborate on the development, delivery, and evaluation of courses. The degree of involvement or direction of any one discipline varies according to the model selected. Curriculum development, implementation, and evaluation of multi-, inter-, and transdisciplinary models depend largely on faculty commitment to the goal of better understanding of multiple roles, fostering inter-professional relationships, and acknowledging the contributions of each discipline. Dyer (2003) has summarized the different models.

A *multidisciplinary model* is one in which a single discipline-specific faculty member determines which additional disciplines should be involved in providing the goals and resources relevant for student learning. In this way, a specific course is taught by a faculty member from one discipline, while recognizing and helping all participating students achieve goals critical to their specific disciplines.

The interdisciplinary model requires greater collaboration and interdependence among team members from relevant disciplines. In this model, members from the collaborating disciplines take responsibility for jointly planning, developing, and teaching portions of the course for which they are expert, to students from the participating disciplines.

Transdisciplinary models require a different degree of team sharing and collaboration. In course development and delivery, expertise from different disciplines is shared across these disciplines. Concepts and processes are integrated. Boundary blurring occurs, as well as mutual trust and respect for discipline-specific expertise. For example, a transdisciplinary curriculum with an organizing framework of roles could include both core transdisciplinary and discipline-specific features for the roles of care provider/patient advocate, collaborator, leader, and researcher (Massey, 2001).

Ordering of Knowledge

Wiles and Bondi (1998) describe five ways of ordering knowledge in a curriculum:

- *building blocks*: essential components are identified and sequenced and deviation is not allowed
- *branching*: foundational components are required and choices are given for higher-level learning
- *spiral*: the same content area is repeatedly revisited at higher levels of complexity
- *skills* (or *competency*): ordering of content is flexible
- *process*: a fluid organization of knowledge is possible since content is the medium through which specified processes are addressed

Nursing curricula with course choices (i.e., branching), would reflect a belief that there is more than one path to reach the goals. Many programs have a final practicum and this experience provides an example of both branching and spiraling. A variety of placements for a practicum represent a branching design. Students who repeat a placement they have previously experienced are in a spiral situation: they are returning to the same practice area with more knowledge and experience.

Course Sequencing Patterns

Within the organizing strategy used to design the curriculum, courses can be sequenced in *block* or *concurrent patterns*. A *block pattern* specifies theory courses and clinical experiences in sequence, each separate from the other and becoming the foundation for those that follow. A *concurrent pattern* specifies that theory courses and clinical experiences are scheduled simultaneously throughout the curriculum.

A *mixed pattern* is also possible, with different parts of the curriculum having different patterns. A program with concurrent theory and practice, followed by a concentrated clinical practicum without formal classes, is an example of a mixed pattern for sequencing learning experiences.

Curriculum Design Process

Creating a curriculum design involves many processes. These include defining curriculum parameters; deliberating about delivery approaches, program models, organizing strategies, and course sequencing; identifying courses; and attending to program policies and resources. Iterative discussions lead to the generation of design proposals, critique, and decision-making. There is no formula for curriculum design, such that a particular model and organizing strategy results in a pre-determined design. Each design team will establish its own procedures, and through the use of both creative and logical thinking, produce a design that is relevant for its own circumstances. Invariably, the design group's work will be characterized by ongoing deliberation and negotiation.

Defining Curriculum Parameters

Attention to curriculum design, i.e., the configuration of the program of studies, cannot occur in isolation of contextual data. The design is affected by realities over which curricularists may have little or no influence. These are the parameters within which the design must be created. Additionally, contextual data and all curriculum decisions made thus far will make some designs possible, while ruling out others. Therefore, it is worthwhile for members of the design subcommittee to review and clarify the parameters that will affect the design in their school.

A review of contextual data can highlight relevant information that curriculum designers must keep in mind. Internal data might include faculty numbers, infrastructure, institutional policies, partnerships, commitment to distance education, and the ability of other departments to mount new courses. Critical data from the external environment include standards and criteria for national accreditation, and approval by state or provincial nursing organizations.

It is important for curriculum designers to be clear about these parameters, so that a realistic and feasible curriculum will be created. The goal is to design a curriculum that:

- is congruent with agreed-upon philosophical approaches
- creates opportunities for students to achieve curriculum goals

- is responsive to the context in which it will be operationalized
- will meet requirements for accreditation
- will be supported by the educational institution

Facilitating the Design Process

Designing the curriculum, which requires time and considerable intellectual effort, can be facilitated by reviewing current literature, visiting other schools, consulting with colleagues regionally and nationally, and attending nursing education conferences. Surveys of catalogues of highly rated schools (particularly those using similar philosophical approaches), with attention to program designs, could prove beneficial and move the process forward.

To solicit input, the design team could develop a template and ask stakeholders to respond to the designated elements. Following statements about the philosophical approaches and curriculum goals, the template could include space for year goals, semester goals, possible courses, credit allocations, sequencing, clinical experiences, and other items deemed relevant. The collation of this information can provide a basis for curriculum design. As well, assistance from an expert in curriculum design could be profitable to provide ideas about possible designs.

A two-dimensional grid or matrix is another way to facilitate the design process (Heinrich, Karner, Gaglione, & Lambert, 2002). The grid, with pertinent horizontal and vertical headings, can be useful to illustrate the emerging curriculum. A somewhat older, but "tried and true" tool, it would indicate:

- interrelationships among concepts
- content links between and among courses
- gaps and redundancies in the knowledge base, experiences, or skills

See Table 8.1 for an example of a matrix.

Deliberating About Curriculum Design

Deliberations about curriculum design encompass integrative discussion about all aspects of design as well as focused discussion about the specific components of design. The overall purpose is to create the configuration of the program of studies. Therefore, dialogue could center around the following questions.

- How can the philosophical approaches be operationalized?
- How can the curriculum be designed so students will have opportunities to achieve the curriculum goals?
- Will distance delivery, on-campus classes, or a combination be used?
- What could the program model be?

TABLE 8.1   EXAMPLE OF MATRIX SHOWING CURRICULUM CONCEPTS IN COURSES

Nursing Courses	Curriculum Concepts				
	Health promotion	Caring for diverse clients	Professionalism	Interpersonal collaboration	Nursing knowledge and competence
The Nursing Profession		✓	✓	✓	✓
Nursing of Families	✓	✓	✓	✓	✓
Nursing Care in Episodic Illness	✓	✓	✓	✓	✓
Transcultural Nursing	✓	✓	✓	✓	✓
Nursing Research			✓		✓

- What could be the overall organizing strategy for the design?
- Which pattern for sequencing learning experiences matches our beliefs about learning?
- What are the learning experiences (theory and practice) that students require to achieve curriculum goals?
- Which are the necessary nursing and support courses?
- Which courses could be multi-, inter-, or trans-disciplinary?
- Which courses could be optional for students?
- What configurations of courses are possible to maximize learning?
- What is the rationale for the delivery approach, model, organizing strategy, and configuration chosen?
- What academic policies should be considered as part of the design?

Some design elements are addressed in detail below. Notably, these include selecting delivery approaches, a program model, an organizing strategy, and course-sequencing pattern.

Selecting a Delivery Approach Decisions about delivery (face-to-face or distance) form an important part of the overall discussion, if this has not already been defined as a parameter. Referring to contextual data about faculty, institutional support for distance education, and available infrastructure, designers might ask:

- Is the use of only one delivery approach congruent with philosophical approaches and curriculum goals, or should a combination be used?
- Which modalities would best suit the nature of the curriculum?
- What resources would faculty require?
- What resources will students require for distance education (e.g., personal computers, access to video-conferencing facilities)?
- How might delivery approaches affect the configuration of courses?

Selecting a Program Model   When curriculum designers have the option of creating a new program model, their deliberations are strongly guided by beliefs about learning. They can ask themselves:

- Which arrangement of nursing and support courses best match the philosophical approaches, curriculum goals, and faculty beliefs about learning?
- Which arrangements can be ruled out?
- Which model will be feasible and acceptable to students, faculty, and the educational institution?

Selecting an Organizing Strategy and a Course-Sequencing Pattern   The choice of an organizing strategy will depend on the philosophical approaches previously determined for the curriculum and the concepts identified as being important (see Chapters 6 and 7). Stakeholders working on design might ask themselves questions such as:

- What are appropriate criteria for choosing an organizing strategy and sequencing pattern?
- Which organizing strategies can be ruled out?
- Which organizing strategies might fit with the philosophical approaches?
- Do faculty support one theory of nursing, pluralism, or eclecticism?
- Is there a natural fit with curriculum concepts and one of the organizing strategies?
- Can some of the organizing strategies be combined in a meaningful way?
- Should a block, concurrent, or mixed pattern of course sequencing be used?

These, and other points of discussion, will lead to a conclusion about an organizing strategy and sequencing pattern. Like all aspects of curriculum development, the process is iterative, with ideas being proposed and, following debate and review of previous decisions, modifications made and new ideas added.

Identifying Courses

Discussion about courses to include in the curriculum requires attention to many ideas concurrently. The *scope and depth* (i.e., what is to be learned), the *sequence* (progression from one unit to another), and *continuity* (relationships among learnings) are significant concerns for curriculum designers. The balance between content and process can be a source of much deliberation, possibly reflecting differing values in the group.

Identifying appropriate courses begins with an examination of the curriculum goals, followed by discussion about pre-requisite knowledge and experiences (Boland, 2005; Gagné, Briggs, & Wager, 1992). Recognition of courses that are not suitable occurs as part of the discussion and helps to define which ideas are relevant. The pre-requisite knowledge and experiences form the basis of nursing and non-nursing courses.

Typically, the curriculum goals are those for the graduating year or final semester of the program. Working backward from these, year or semester goals are identified and then analyzed to form goals for the nursing courses. In this way, the link between individual units of learning (courses) and the curriculum goals are evident. An example of leveling of one curriculum goal for a four-year, baccalaureate-nursing program is given in Table 8.2. Further refinement is required for individual courses (see Chapter 9). Although this approach to curriculum planning is currently most closely identified with an *outcomes* design, it has long been used (Friesner, 1978; Gagné, Briggs, & Wager, 1992; Tyler, 1949).

Nursing Courses   Nursing courses are typically defined first. The interface between goals and the organization of identified concepts gives rise to decisions about the nature, number, and configuration of nursing courses. These decisions rest upon the program model, structure, organizing strategy, course sequencing pattern, and all previous decisions about the curriculum. A review of curriculum concepts and possibilities (see Chapter 6) provides a base for planning. As well, curriculum designers should consider whether courses in other disciplines would be suitable instead of developing a nursing course. The following questions could shape the dialogue.

- Is there a logical grouping of the concepts?
- Which concepts should be incorporated with increasing depth throughout the curriculum?
- How can the identified concepts be organized in the curriculum?
- How could particular concepts fit into particular courses?
- Which ideas about curriculum possibilities should be developed?
- How many nursing courses are possible within the program structure?
- Which nursing courses could be included?
- What will be the overall goals for the identified courses?

TABLE 8.2   EXAMPLE OF LEVELING ONE CURRICULUM GOAL IN A FOUR-YEAR BACCALAUREATE CURRICULUM

Curriculum and Year 4 Goal	Practice evidence-based nursing competently, incorporating best practice guidelines, health promotion perspectives and respect for the diversity and culture of individuals, families, and communities
Year 3 Goals	1. Critique evidence for nursing practice and health promotion 2. Practice health promotion and provide nursing care that is responsive to the diversity and culture of families and communities
Year 2 Goals	1. Assess intercultural components of health care situations and interactions with clients 2. Articulate evidence and rationale for nursing care and health promotion of individuals and families prospectively 3. Provide nursing care and promote the health of individuals and families, taking into account their cultural beliefs, values, and practices
Year 1 Goals	1. Examine evidence for nursing care of individuals and families 2. Base nursing care on rationale from biopsychosocial and nursing sciences 3. Demonstrate respect in interactions with peers, colleagues, and clients

- How will the overall focus of each course contribute to curriculum goals?
- What is a reasonable sequence for these courses?

In defining the general substance of each course, curriculum designers struggle with the tension between essential knowledge for nursing and adherence to curriculum goals and philosophical approaches. If committed to a philosophical approach that includes constructivism, "the challenge for nurse educators is to . . . overcome the focus on covering content at the expense of engaging students in thinking" (Ironside, 2004, p.6). This challenge exists when first describing each course, and later when planning and implementing courses.

Although course details will be defined later (see Chapter 9), at this time it is important to be clear about the general focus of each course. Titles given to the nursing courses should match the philosophical approaches, curriculum directions, and goals, since the nomenclature gives both conceptual and visual unity to the curriculum. Brief course descriptions and overall course goals should be drafted so that all members of the curriculum development team have an understanding of the intent of each course. These descriptions and goals will be refined and further delineated as detailed course planning proceeds and the links among courses are examined more closely.

Use of a curriculum matrix can ensure that essential concepts and courses are included in the design. The matrix is a visual plan for continuity and increasing depth of concepts, not a detailed summary of the entire curriculum. Rather, it is a recording of prominent ideas for each nursing course and the basis for detailed course planning (see Chapter 9) and evaluation planning (see Chapter 10). Subsequently, when courses are developed, they can be compared to the matrix and to each other to ensure that important elements are present.

Support Courses   Consideration is given to support courses that also contribute to students' knowledge and understanding of the discipline. Substantive knowledge from liberal arts and psychosocial and health sciences is integral to the development of open-minded, educated, and informed practitioners. Students' interaction with an array of concepts, processes, and worldviews expands the depth and scope of their learning, and helps them to think critically from a broader, more comprehensive knowledge base.

Thought is given to which support courses to include, their pre-requisites, modifications to existing courses, or development of new courses. This is accomplished through discussion about the nature of the courses, their fit in the curriculum, and how they support and extend achievement of curriculum goals.

Multi-Inter-Trans-Disciplinary Courses   Courses shared across health science disciplines can form part of the curriculum as elective or required classroom or clinical courses. Since it is important for nursing students to respect the goals and perspectives of other disciplines, and learn to work collaboratively with members of many health disciplines, they should be provided with opportunities to learn in varied disciplinary teams and practice settings. Faculty committed to *interdisciplinary* education and practice in particular should design and schedule courses in concert with faculty from other disciplines, bearing in mind each discipline's curriculum goals, philosophies, and interdependent roles. Intellectual cross-pollination among students should be a constant feature of courses through discussion, projects, and shared clinical learning. For interdisciplinary clinical experiences, faculty must obtain suitable clinical facilities and arrange experiences for each discipline. Interdisciplinary conferences would be necessary to meet established goals. Inclusion of *transdisciplinary* courses in the emerging nursing curriculum design would help meet goals related to effective functioning in *multidisciplinary* environments (Cloonan, Davis, & Burnett, 1999; Gelmon, White, Carlson, & Norman, 2000).

Elective Courses   Elective or optional courses, both within and outside of nursing, can be a valuable component of the curriculum design. The purpose of elective courses is to provide students with opportunities to meet personal learning goals and support the freedom to explore interests in nursing and other disciplines. The design team may require electives at a specific academic level or from particular disciplines. Conversely, faculty may believe that students should choose elective courses freely, without constraint. These decisions will hinge on philosophical approaches and curriculum goals.

Determining Policies and Guidelines

Developing new policies, or modifying existing ones, is part of the curriculum design process. A policy is a firm course of action that must be adhered to in every situation (e.g., appeals policy). The function of policies is to support and guide the achievement of the program and institutional mission and goals (Applegate, 1998). When devising policies, curriculum designers should differentiate between policies and less formal guidelines for action. Guidelines, or guiding principles, present an appropriate course of action for a specific situation, although there may be some context-dependent flexibility (e.g., dress code).

Some policies will be in place within the educational institution and apply to all academic constituencies, while others will be discipline-specific. The latter must be congruent with those of the larger institution, as well as with philosophical approaches of the curriculum. Policies must be readily available to all members of the academic community so that the "rules" are known. The number and nature of policies will vary among nursing programs. Nevertheless, there are some fundamental matters about which policies will be evident in all programs. The following are examples:

- *Admissions and Progressions:* Admissions policies state the criteria used to determine whether an applicant meets admission standards. Progressions policies address advancement in the program, specifically the requirements to progress to subsequent years or semesters. These normally include statements about passing grades for classroom and clinical courses, required grade point average, and whether failing courses can be repeated.

- *Academic Rights and Responsibilities:* Academic rights and responsibilities include, among others, an Appeals Policy and a Code of Student Conduct. An appeal is a formal request by a student to have an academic decision about a grade or adherence to a policy reviewed and changed. Normally, the institution will have a formal process for students and faculty to follow. A Code of Student Conduct outlines what is viewed as acceptable behavior in the institution and may be an example of a policy with more flexibility than an admission policy.

Other policies and guidelines can be formulated specifically for the nursing program, such as attendance (clinical, laboratories, and/or class), definition and consequences of unsafe clinical practice, immunization, language proficiency standards, and dress code. Additional institutional policies can include those related to scholastic discipline, student support, enrollment status, graduation requirements, non-discrimination, and human rights.

Considering Human and Financial Implications

Each curriculum has human and financial implications, and therefore, the curriculum leader should keep the dean or director informed of the emerging design. A successful design depends on the availability of adequate resources for implementation, and the school leader is in the best position to know if those resources will be present.

If, for example, the new curriculum includes more nursing courses than previously, or more clinical practice time, there will be increased teaching costs. The dean or director knows if the school can afford this and whether faculty recruitment should be initiated. If financial resources in the school cannot support the proposed design, then the school leader knows how and with whom to negotiate for additional funding. Modifications to the design will be necessary if adequate financial resources are not forthcoming.

Alternately, a curriculum change may mean that some faculty will no longer be required. A change from supervised clinical practice to more independent practice, for example, could result in reduced numbers of clinical faculty. The dean or director may need to inform longstanding part-time clinical faculty that their employment will be decreased in amount or cease entirely. Concomitant with decreased faculty costs could be a decreased budget for the school. If so, the school leader will have to strategize to retain the school's budget.

A new curriculum design might mean significantly changed teaching assignments for some faculty. Again, the school leader needs to be fully apprised of the emerging design so that teaching assignments and faculty development can be planned.

A curriculum change can have financial implications for students and this should be taken into account when designing a curriculum. An increased reliance on distance delivery could make it possible for geographically dispersed students to enroll in the nursing program. Yet, if those students must then travel a considerable distance for clinical experience, the associated costs could preclude their enrollment. Similarly, on-campus students may find travel to new practice sites difficult. It is important that the anticipated costs to students be considered and that accurate information be provided to prospective students.

Deciding on the Design

When deciding on a curriculum design, developers should probably construct several designs, with different configurations of courses, and judge the advantages and disadvantages of each. The one selected should be optimally useful, consistent and appropriate, responsive to current and future social contexts, flexible enough to allow for future refinement, and congruent with the philosophical approaches selected for the curriculum.

Like other aspects of curriculum development, the design subcommittee's work must be reviewed and approved by the Total Faculty Group. The subcommittee presents the configuration of courses, year or semester goals, course goals, and brief course descriptions to the total faculty. Inclusion of the matrix or template can facilitate the group's understanding.

Summary of Curriculum Design Process

The complex process of curriculum design cannot be accurately described in a formulaic manner. Faculty must be cognizant of the parameters in which the curriculum will be operationalized so their efforts are directed toward the creation of a curriculum that will be supported by the school and educational institution. Existing parameters (such as the program structure, partnership, commitments about delivery approaches) affect all deliberations and decisions. Decisions about an organizing strategy for design, program model, courses and their sequencing, and so forth, must be congruent with curriculum goals and philosophical approaches. Discussion is iterative and integrative, with ideas about curriculum design emerging for critique, negotiation, development, and decision.

Faculty Development

The overall goal of faculty development in relation to curriculum design is to expand members' appreciation and knowledge of curriculum design. As with all aspects of faculty development, the precise activities will be dependent on the needs of faculty.

Faculty development can include a brief review of parameters as a reminder that a feasible curriculum is the goal. Then, attention can be given to the process of curriculum design and possible configurations of courses that could be congruent with the philosophical approaches and curriculum goals. In a workshop setting, a template might be introduced for small groups to complete. The completed templates could then be given to the design team for consideration. In this way, the faculty development activity contributes directly to the design process.

An additional activity would be to introduce a curriculum matrix, with course names and concepts identified. Workshop participants could complete the matrix, which would help them understand the inter-relatedness of concepts and design possibilities. Those members with expertise in curriculum development can readily facilitate these activities.

Chapter Summary

The curriculum design is the configuration of the program of studies. The design must be congruent with the institution and school's mission and purpose, and with the faculty's values and beliefs. It should be directed and oriented to student learning, and reflect the philosophical approaches, goals, and context of nursing. Curriculum developers should have a clear sense of purpose and commitment to completing the task of design. Because of the human and financial implications, the school leader must be apprised of the emerging design.

The chapter includes descriptions of elements important in curriculum design such as partnerships, delivery approaches, curriculum models, organizing strategies, and patterns for course sequencing. The process of designing curricula is detailed, beginning with acknowledging the curriculum parameters; selecting delivery approaches, program model, and organizing strategies; and identifying courses. Policy development is addressed, as are human and financial implications of curriculum design.

Synthesis Activities

Below are two case studies. The Van-Buren University case is followed by a critique. Discuss the case and its analysis, considering additional ideas that arise. The second, Fitzhugh University, is followed by questions to guide examination of the case. Questions to assist in curriculum design follow.

Van-Buren University

Van-Buren is a small private university in southern California, well known for its creativity and progressive thinking in all aspects of academic life. The school of nursing and school of medicine have a long history of collaboration and several core courses are shared. Over the last three years, the deans of both schools noted numerous requests from alumni for a program focused on non-traditional health and healing.

Following several joint faculty meetings, a curriculum committee was formed with faculty volunteers and alumni representing both schools and other stakeholders. They worked on developing a curriculum to respond to alumni requests. They also discussed possible courses, delivery approaches, and practice placements. The curriculum committee surveyed their colleagues' ideas and reviewed calendars of many existing programs in complementary therapies, including some in Europe and Asia. As well, two 1-hour videoconferenced faculty development sessions were held with consultants from existing programs, to learn about successes and challenges. These discussions generated interest about exploring future reciprocal practice placements.

Task forces were then created and their collective work culminated in a decision to support the development of an interdisciplinary, continuing-education certificate program in complementary health and healing practices to promote wellness and stress reduction. Consensus was also achieved about adopting a holistic, client-centered philosophical approach. Both deans agreed that the resources needed to develop, support, and offer the curriculum would be shared equally, as would the tuitions generated.

Faculty members in each school were asked to respond to draft curriculum goals and prioritize the curriculum concepts that were suggested in previous brainstorming discussions. They were also asked to propose course delivery methods and possible clinical experiences. The committee then synthesized the data, and drafted brief course descriptions and a curriculum matrix that included courses and concepts given highest priority by faculty. A blend of video- and computer-conferencing technologies was proposed for course delivery.

Critique It is evident that faculty from both schools have a history of working together and value interdisciplinary education and practice. The curriculum committee is working hard to ensure that faculty supports the evolving program design. Seeking faculty input through discussions, surveys, and responses to the matrix are strengths of the design process and should promote program ownership. Integrating faculty-development sessions early in the process heightened interest, commitment to innovation, and cross-cultural networking and partnership potential. As well, issues related to program goals, length, and delivery approach were settled early.

Faculty should now decide whether the course titles and core concepts capture the ideas they proposed. They should also consider whether students ought to have experience in more than one therapeutic modality during the practicum. Decisions about whether the certificate courses would be credit or non-credit, the length of each course, how the courses will be developed, who will teach them, and if courses would be offered concurrently or sequentially still need to be determined.

Fitzhugh University

Fitzhugh University is an accredited university of approximately 16,000 full-time and 8,400 part-time students, offering baccalaureate, masters, and doctoral arts and science programs. It is located in a multicultural city of 780,000 inhabitants. Potential practice facilities for nursing students are numerous. Nursing students have access to three acute care hospitals, one of which is a 450-bed magnet hospital; two community health care agencies; three chronic and long-term care facilities; many schools (nursery, K-7, middle and high school); industry; as well as physician offices and walk-in clinics.

The nursing faculty, which comprises 20 masters-prepared and 5 doctorally-prepared members, has been meeting regularly for six months to completely redesign their baccalaureate program. The goal is to implement the revised curriculum in 18 months for a class of 75 students.

The curriculum committee, with consensus from the entire faculty, has determined curriculum directions for the revised curriculum based on the existing humanistic-caring philosophical approach. Recently, in order to obtain design ideas, some members visited several schools of nursing offering 'state-of-the-art' baccalaureate nursing programs, while other committee members reviewed current literature and catalogues of accredited nursing programs. The curriculum committee is influenced by National League for Nursing reforms and, accordingly, has decided to use an outcomes approach for the curriculum design.

Dr. Helena Trakopolous, the school director, has consistently supported the curriculum committee's decisions and endorses the outcome design. She reminds faculty to be cognizant of the university's mission, the school's philosophical approaches and goals, current nursing and health care trends, and the learning needs of students.

The curriculum committee has produced a list of agreed-upon outcomes and competencies for graduates of the new program. These include safe practice in health care settings, critical thinking, effective communication and management, ethical and cultural competence, and legal and political awareness. The curriculum coordinator has called another meeting, the purpose of which is to identify the work yet to be done. On the agenda is how to distinguish outcomes from competencies, how to write them, and how to discern their relationships. Leveling of competencies according to year and semester of the program, the practice context for each semester, and the core knowledge upon which the curriculum will be based will also be discussed.

Questions for Consideration and Analysis of the Fitzhugh University Case

1. How should the curriculum committee proceed with the work yet to be done?
2. What should the curriculum committee consider next?
3. What resources would assist the committee in its design activities?
4. What should be included in the curriculum design?
5. How could nursing and non-nursing courses be determined?
6. What policies should be taken into account for the curriculum design?
7. Draft a curriculum matrix for outcomes, competencies, and core knowledge that could be included in the curriculum design.

Curriculum Development Activities for Consideration in Your Setting

Use the following questions to guide thinking about designing your curriculum.

1. Which program structure is most appropriate for the type of program we are developing?

2. Which program model most clearly reflects our beliefs about learning?

3. How do our partnerships and delivery methods influence the design?

4. What organizing strategy might we select to assure a logical progression to, and achievement of, curriculum goals?

5. What should we include in the curriculum matrix?

6. What nursing, support, and elective courses will best facilitate achievement of program goals? Should there be inter-, multi-, or transdisciplinary courses?

7. What configuration of courses should be considered?

8. How can courses be titled to ensure conceptual unity?

9. What negotiations should take place with other academic units to operationalize the envisioned curriculum?

10. Which existing institutional policies influence our design?

11. Which specific policies need to be developed?

12. What are the resource implications of our curriculum design?

13. What approaches might be considered to enhance faculty understanding about, and commitment to, the curriculum design?

References

Andrusyszyn, M.A. (1998). *Instructor's guide to computer conferencing.* Retrieved February 18, 2004 from http://publish.uwo.ca/~maandrus/cmcgui~1.htm

Applegate, M.A. (1998). Educational program evaluation. In D.M. Billings & J.A. Halstead (Eds.), *Teaching in nursing. A guide for faculty.* (pp. 423–457). Philadelphia: W. B. Saunders Co.

Arthur, H., & Baumann, A. (1996). Nursing curriculum content: An innovative decision-making process to define priorities. *Nurse Education Today, 16,* 63–68.

Bayliss-Webber, P. (2002). A curriculum framework for nursing. *Journal of Nursing Education, 41*(1), 15–24.

Boland, D.L. (1998). Developing curriculum frameworks, outcomes and competencies. In D.M. Billings & J.A. Halstead (Eds.), *Teaching in nursing. A guide for faculty.* (pp. 135–150). Philadelphia: W. B. Saunders Co.

Boland, D.L. (2005). Developing curriculum frameworks, outcomes and competencies. In D.M. Billings & J.A. Halstead (Eds.), *Teaching in nursing. A guide for faculty* (2nd ed.). (pp. 167–185). St. Louis: Elsevier Saunders.

Bowen, M., Lyons, K.J., & Young, B.E. (2000). Nursing and health care reform. Implications for curriculum development. *Journal of Nursing Education, 39*(1), 27–33.

Burge, E., & Roberts, J.M. (1993). *Classrooms with a difference: A practical guide to the use of conferencing technologies.* Toronto: Distance Learning Office Field Services and Research, The Ontario Institute for Studies in Education.

Cloonan, P.A., Davis, F.D., & Burnett, C. B. (1999). Interdisciplinary education in clinical ethics: A work in progress. *Holistic Nursing Practice, 13*(2), 12–19.

Dyer, J. (2003). Multidisciplinary, interdisciplinary, and transdisciplinary educational models and nursing education. *Nursing Education Perspectives, 24*(4), 186–188.

Eckhardt, J.A., Mathias Anderson, D., Campbell, S.E., Clarke, S.E., & Pavlish, C.L. (2002). A theoretical framework for RN to BSN education. *Nursing Education Perspectives, 23*(3), 124–127.

Freeman, L.H., Voignier, R.R., & Scott, D.L. (2002). New curriculum for a new century: Beyond repackaging. *Nursing Education Perspectives, 23*(1), 38–40.

Friesner, A. (1978). Curriculum process for developing or revising a baccalaureate nursing program. (pp. 13–22). In NLN. *Curriculum process for developing or revising a baccalaureate nursing program.* New York: Author.

Gagné, R.M., Briggs, L.J., & Wager, W.W. (1992). *Principles of instructional design.* (4th ed.). Fort Worth: Harcourt Brace Jovanovich College Publishers.

Gelmon, S.B., White, A.W., Carlson, L., & Norman, L. (2000). Making organizational change to achieve improvements and interprofessional learning: perspectives from health professions educators. *Journal of Interprofessional Care, 14*(2), 131–146.

Gubrud-Howe, P., Shaver, K.S., Tanner, C.A., Bennett-Stillmaker, J., Davidson, S.B., Flaherty-Robb, M., et al. (2003). A challenge to meet the future: Nursing education in Oregon, 2010. *Journal of Nursing Education, 42*(4), 163–167.

Harasim, L., Hiltz, S.R., Teles, L., & Turoff, M. (1995). *Learning networks: A field guide to teaching and learning online.* Cambridge, MA: The MIT Press.

Heinrich, C.R., Karner, K.J., Gaglione, B.H., & Lambert, L.J. (2002). Order out of chaos. The use of a matrix to validate curriculum integrity. *Nurse Educator, 27*(3), 136–140.

Ironside, P.M. (2004). "Covering content" and teaching thinking: Deconstructing the additive curriculum. *Journal of Nursing Education, 43*(1), 5–12.

Lindeman, C.A. (2000). The future of nursing education. *Journal of Nursing Education, 39*(1), 5–12.

Massey, C.M. (2001). A transdisciplinary model for curricular revision. *Nursing Education Perspectives, 22*(2), 85–88.

National League for Nursing. (1993). *A vision for nursing education.* New York: Author.

NLNAC. (2003). *Accreditation Manual for post-secondary and higher degree programs in nursing.* New York: Author.

Pennington, E.A. (1986). The integrated curriculum: A 15-year perspective. In E.A. Pennington (Ed.), *Curriculum revisited: An update of curriculum design.* (pp. 37–48). New York: National League for Nursing.

Picciano, A.G. (2001*). Distance learning: Making connection across virtual space and time.* Upper Saddle River, NJ: Prentice-Hall.

Shiber, S. (2003). A nursing education model for second-degree students. *Nursing Education Perspectives, 24,* 124–138.

Tyler, R.M. (1949). *Basic Principles of curriculum and instruction.* Chicago: The University of Chicago Press.

Wiles, J., & Bondi, J. (1998). *Curriculum development: A guide to practice.* Upper Saddle River, NJ: Merrill.

CHAPTER 9

Course Design

Chapter Overview

Following completion of the curriculum design, attention turns to the design of individual courses. In this chapter, descriptions of course components and design parameters are followed by approaches to course design. Consideration is given to designing distance courses. A brief overview of teaching strategies is presented. The process of course design is detailed, followed by ideas about designing individual classes and possible activities for faculty development. The chapter concludes with a summary and synthesis activities.

Chapter Goals

- Identify course components
- Consider parameters influencing course design
- Examine approaches to course design
- Understand the process of course design
- Reflect on faculty development activities to facilitate course design

Course Design

An academic course is a recognized unit of learning within an overall curriculum. It is designed with components that outline what is to be taught, learned, and evaluated. The intent of course design is to achieve unity and coherence within each course and among courses.

Course design begins as soon as a curriculum design has been approved, and truly never ends, since courses are refined throughout the life of the curriculum. It is a cyclical process: after implementation, courses are evaluated and designs modified.

The term *course design*, when used as a noun, refers to the configuration of a course. The design encompasses all components (purpose, goals, teaching and evaluation strategies, content, classes, and learning activities), and the relationships between and among them. The *process of designing courses*, or the *course design process*, refers to discussions and decision-making that lead to the configuration of a course. The course design process personalizes the impending curriculum change since faculty members feel a sense of ownership about the courses they create and teach.

Course design proceeds once the curriculum design is approved. The level goals, brief course descriptions, and overall course goals developed during curriculum design become the starting point for designing courses. The philosophical approaches and goals approved for the curriculum are realized within courses.

The terminology used to describe course components varies among nursing programs. Nonetheless, the components of purpose, goals, teaching and evaluation strategies, content, classes, and learning activities are present in all academic courses, whether they are classroom, clinical, laboratory, or distance.

Course Components

Purpose and Description

All courses have a purpose in a nursing curriculum. A statement of purpose makes evident why the course is part of the curriculum and how it contributes to students' achievement of curriculum goals. Although the purpose may be readily apparent to curriculum designers, the reason for the course might not be obvious to students. An explicit statement of purpose can orient students to the value of the course in their learning.

Each course requires a brief description that is published in the institutional catalogue or calendar. This description is expanded in course materials to be meaningful for students enrolled in the course. It provides information about the scope of the course, preparation required for classes, the nature of class meetings, participation expected of students, and other information that faculty consider important to explain the intent and character of the course. Class or clinical hours and course credits are generally stated. Table 9.1 is an example of a course purpose and expanded description.

Course Goals

Goals are another component of courses. Learning, a process that leads to the acquisition of new knowledge, understanding, and abilities, is the ultimate purpose for which courses

TABLE 9.1   PURPOSE AND DESCRIPTION OF A JUNIOR LEVEL BACCALAUREATE COURSE

Nursing 376 Teaching and Learning in Nursing Practice

The purposes of this course are to expand students' a) understanding of the processes of teaching and learning in nursing practice, and b) skill in assessing health learning needs, providing health information that is meaningful to clients, and evaluating learning. Successful completion of this course will contribute to the following curriculum goals:

- Practice evidence-based, competent nursing, incorporating best practice guidelines, health promotion perspectives, and respect for the diversity and culture of individuals, families, and communities
- Demonstrate leadership in planning, providing, managing, and evaluating care in institutional and community settings

Learning gained in this course will contribute to practice in all areas of nursing, and to students' appreciation of their own learning processes.

In this course, students will explore the role of the nurse as teacher and learner in a variety of contexts. Educational theories for teaching, learning, and motivation for health behavior change will be addressed. Concepts and processes involved in teaching and learning are included. Workshops, group presentations and projects, and dialogue about clinical practice will provide opportunities to integrate theory and practice. Preparation and active participation is integral to all classes. 3 hours per week, 13 weeks. 3 credits

are designed. The nature of the desired learning is evident in the course goals. General course goals, derived from curriculum and year or semester goals, are formulated when courses are identified and configured as part of curriculum design (Chapter 8). These general goals must be refined to make them specific for the course. Course goals describe the abilities or competencies expected of students at the end of the course and are written in the same format as overall curriculum goals.

Course goals state the expected competencies in relevant learning domains. As well, important concepts for the course can be included in the goal statements. Typically, the number of goals exceeds those delineated for each semester because the expectations for courses are more explicit. Table 9.2 presents examples of how the same semester goal can be individualized for two different courses.

Teaching Strategies

Teaching strategies are the actions employed by an instructor to facilitate students' achievement of learning goals, namely the development of abilities necessary to practice professional

TABLE 9.2   EXAMPLE OF COURSE GOALS RELATED TO THE SAME SEMESTER GOAL

SEMESTER GOAL: Practice evidence-based nursing, demonstrating respect for diversity of clients

Courses	Course Goals
Teaching and Learning in Nursing	1. Critically examine a variety of educational and health-behavior theories
	2. Develop and implement practical approaches to facilitate learning of clients with a diversity of ages, cultures, and health concerns
Health Promotion of Community Groups	1. Assess beliefs and practices associated with emotional and physical well-being of selected groups
	2. Plan and implement health-promoting interventions that reflect current health promotion research and respect for group beliefs and values

nursing competently. The strategies selected should be congruent with the curriculum's philosophical approaches, and should assist students in meeting course goals.

Course Content

The course content is the component that can be of most interest to students who want to know what they need to learn. The scope of content is specified for each course, and in classroom courses, this typically is conveyed to students in the form of titles or topics for each class meeting, along with a list of required readings.

Courses contain substantive knowledge (facts, concepts, hypotheses, methods, to name a few) through which the thinking processes for nursing practice are developed. No matter how the information is addressed, each course has content. The content must be judiciously selected, with only the most pertinent chosen.

In courses where faculty are most concerned with students' engagement with content, that is, creating meaning and discerning its significance to practice (Ironside, 2004), the content is still important. Even though processing of information is primary, the basic issue of identifying suitable content remains.

Content in clinical courses is the knowledge required to practice in designated clinical situations, the knowledge and skills (cognitive, psychomotor, affective) developed, and the clinical situations themselves. Being in the situation, applying previously held and new knowledge and abilities, seeking learning opportunities, and formulating new understandings are the intent of clinical courses. Therefore, a weekly topical schedule is not applicable.

Classes

Each course has a specified number and duration of formal sessions when faculty and students interact. These sessions can be conducted in classrooms, clinical settings, labs, or online. In classroom courses, typically a topic is identified for each session. Although the structure of online courses may vary, they generally retain the idea of a "class" in which a conceptually meaningful unit of content is addressed. For clinical or laboratory courses, the "class" is each practice session.

Student Learning Activities

Courses include activities planned specifically to provide opportunities for students to process information and work toward achievement of course goals through interaction with course content, faculty, and other students. The planned learning activities can be online interactions, group projects, laboratory and clinical experiences, discussions, and so forth. The key feature of student learning activities is that they require active engagement of learners.

Evaluation of Student Learning

Assessment of student learning is a component of critical interest to students and faculty. Evaluation procedures can include essays, examinations, projects, presentations, journals, clinical performance, etc. Whichever are used, they must be congruent with the philosophical approaches and goals of the curriculum.

Course Design Parameters

There are a number of parameters within which courses are designed. These boundaries limit the range that faculty have in creating courses, yet compel them to exercise creativity and ingenuity in designing courses that are motivating and promote positive learning experiences.

Philosophical Approaches and Curriculum Goals The overriding parameters for all courses are the school's philosophical approaches and curriculum goals. Courses must be congruent with these. Additionally, if the curriculum is being organized according to specified theories, conceptual models, or frameworks, these must be evident in the goals, approach to content, and evaluation of student learning. Importantly, the philosophical approaches influence all learning experiences and evaluation of student learning. They also define the desired learning climate of the course.

Course Level, Structure, and Delivery The level of the course, that is, the semester and year in the program, is a significant parameter of course design. Students' prior learning determines the depth and scope of the course. Course structure (i.e., course length; frequency, duration, and time of sessions) also has a direct bearing on the outcomes to be achieved, the extent of the subject matter, and evaluation. Course delivery approaches determine how students access and engage in the course.

Students' Characteristics The number and characteristics of students in the course influence course design. Attitudes toward learning, technology, participation, and evaluation are important factors. Similarly, students' cultural diversity, maturity, motivation, interests, and other commitments have a bearing on course design.

Physical Environment Desk arrangements, temperature, windows, ventilation, and lighting have an effect on attention, fatigue, and interactions, and must be considered in course design. As well, for clinical courses, the physical setting influences learning opportunities.

Human and Material Resources The numbers of faculty and graduate teaching assistants, and their experiences, affect the decisions that are made about individual courses. Library and computer resources and technical equipment in classrooms, among other material resources, must also be considered.

Policies and Contractual Agreements Finally, the educational institution may have policies or regulations that must be respected in course design. For example, there may be requirements about evaluation and examinations. For clinical courses, contractual arrangements with clinical or community agencies regulate learning experiences.

Approaches to Course Design

The approach to course design is strongly influenced by faculty members' abilities, interests, and comfort level, as well as the background knowledge, life experiences, and capabilities of students. Often, faculty use a familiar approach without giving careful thought to what is congruent with the curriculum goals and philosophical approaches. If this occurs, discussion leading to consensus about an effective overall approach may be necessary. However, some flexibility in approaches to course design may be appropriate.

Irrespective of the approach to course design, attention is given to the diversity of abilities and characteristics of students. Accordingly, course designers strive to ensure that:

- Web sites are readily understandable and intuitive
- opportunities exist for alternate evaluation methods
- written and oral expression is clear and unambiguous
- important ideas receive prominence in course materials
- physical facilities are accessible and comfortable, with good sight lines (Bowe, 2000)

Extending from the idea of making courses intellectually and physically accessible is the belief that courses should be culturally comfortable for students of differing heritages. Therefore, deliberate effort is made to avoid ethnocentric and gender-limited language, texts, readings, and learning experiences. Additionally, authors with varied backgrounds should be represented in course readings (Saunders & Kardia, n.d.). The intent is to make the course as inclusive as possible so all students feel welcome and accepted in an environment conducive to learning.

Traditional Approaches

In traditional approaches to course design, planning proceeds in a logical, step-wise fashion, starting with objectives. The intent is to design a course and lessons that will lead students to learn specific content in a readily identified and prescribed way.

With this approach, a course description is written first. Then, course objectives are formulated according to taxonomies that address cognitive, psychomotor, and affective domains of learning. The course objectives state what the learner will be able to do, think, or feel. They are drawn from program and level objectives, the course description, and content necessary for the desired behaviors to occur. As well, unit or module objectives are specified, with the units being defined by content groupings. "Courses are constructed around the content deemed necessary to produce the desired target behaviors" (Bevis, 1982, p.195). Teaching strategies, media, and evaluation methods are then selected.

Gagné, Briggs, and Wager (1992) propose a more detailed approach, whereby following the specification of program goals, an instructional analysis is completed to identify the skills involved in reaching those goals. This entails a task analysis to delineate the steps or skills in the behavior and an information-processing analysis to identify the mental processes required to enact each goal. From these, objectives are prepared. Next, criterion-referenced evaluation procedures are created and instructional strategies and media selected.

Lesson planning is an important element of traditional approaches. For each lesson, objectives are delineated and appropriate instructional events defined. Written lesson plans specify activities that the teacher will carry out. See Table 9.3 for a sample lesson plan.

The traditional, behaviorist course design is structured, supports knowledge as being absolute, and is teacher-centered. Faculty have responsibility for identifying the nature, purpose, and goals of the course, content, teaching strategies, and evaluation methods. Students are the recipients of knowledge and decisions.

Contemporary Approaches

With a more contemporary or conceptual approach to course design, courses are planned so the focus of learning is on inquiry and the active pursuit of experiences that contribute

TABLE 9.3   LESSON PLAN FOR A 2-HOUR CLASS

Purpose: Provide students with information necessary for health education and promotion

Objectives	Content	Teaching Strategies	Time	Resources	Evaluation Methods
Identify 3 goals of health promotion	Health promotion goals	Lecture-discussion	10 min	Chalk board Overhead or PowerPoint slides	Pre-testing
Describe how the Health Belief Model can be used to influence behavior	Health Belief Model	Lecture-discussion	25 min	PowerPoint slides	Question and answer
Assess concerns of families seeking health promotion interventions	Family health	Case study or role play Discussion	35 min	Guests Discussion questions on over-heads or slides	Question and answer
Recall guidelines for health promotion	Guidelines for health promotion	Brainstorming Large group discussion	20 min	Flip-charts	Question and answer
Examine health promotion measures	Review of course goals	Lecture-discussion	30 min	Questionnaire	Post-testing

to learning. These student-centered course designs incorporate recognition and acceptance of the values, beliefs, knowledge, and experience that learners bring. Courses are designed in accordance with the premises that learning and contextual knowledge:

- evolve from processes such as discussion, dialogue, debate, and other heuristics that promote active engagement and sharing of knowledge
- devolop in an environment of trust that promotes critique among co-learners (teachers and students)

This approach to course design is based on adherence to values of human freedom and self reflection (Watson, 2000), and an epistemology of constructivism. Therefore, course procedures are designed to emphasize students' processing of information and construction of understandings and meanings. Process-oriented courses promote integrative learning, de-emphasize specified content, and reduce reliance on the lecture method of delivering content. Attention is given to how students, faculty, and clients together bring life experiences to knowledge and learning. Understanding develops through thoughtful deliberation and critical analysis of information, dialogue about its meaning, and reflection on its fit with personal beliefs and values (Andrusyszyn, 1998).

Faculty and students share course design, jointly creating the climate and cultural reality in which collaboration flourishes. Together, they determine course goals, and establish appropriate means to meet those goals and to evaluate learning. In this way, students gain a sense of ownership for the course and learning process. They become active constructors of knowledge and meaning (Seaton-Sykes, 2003); they shape their learning through participation in course design and activities. The instructor's role is one of expert learner, metastrategist, and facilitator (Bevis, 2000b), who empowers, fosters creativity, stimulates intellectual inquiry, and requires good scholarship.

Central to contemporary course design is conceptualizing *learning activities*. As stated previously, these enable students to process information and work toward achievement of course goals through interaction with course content, peers, and faculty. They are activities that students undertake with the intent that learning occurs, and can be developed collaboratively, as a part of course design. Learning activities replace instruction; require active involvement and participation; promote self- responsibility for learning; foster synthesis and analysis; and lead to critical thinking, autonomy, personal and professional integrity, and competency (Bevis, 2000a).

Blended Approaches

In a blended approach, there is a mix of contemporary and traditional approaches. In small classes, a contemporary approach may be possible as faculty and student collaboration could occur in all aspects of the course design. In large undergraduate courses, however, some predetermined structure may be required because of class size, agreements with clinical agencies and, perhaps, institutional policies. Therefore, faculty who support constructivism might rely upon an approach to course design that blends both traditional and contemporary perspectives.

Faculty members design the course (i.e., define the description, goals, general scope of content, and evaluation methods) in a way that appears to mirror traditional approaches. Nonetheless, there could be opportunities for student choice within specified limits (Iwasiw, 1987). For example, students may choose from a number of broadly defined assignments or projects and apportion a percentage of the course grade to each.

While courses are designed with a pre-determined structure, their intent is to support process learning. A contemporary approach becomes apparent in the teaching strategies and planned learning activities that occur. For example, planned student activities in lectures (Oermann, 2004), peer teaching (Goldenberg & Iwasiw, 1992; Iwasiw & Goldenberg, 1993), and narrative pedagogy (Diekelmann, 2001; Ironside, 2003), among others, require students to be active participants in learning and knowledge construction. Additionally, faculty can plan guidelines that emphasize process learning in course sessions and make these available to students. The guidelines are student-centered, prepare students for classes, make evident the information processing skills expected, and allow fluidity in the conduct of classes. An example of a class guideline is depicted in Table 9.4. Depending on the nature of the class, specified readings can be included as part of preparatory activities.

Distance Education Approaches

Courses designed for distance education can also incorporate traditional, contemporary, and blended approaches. Key considerations would focus on the opportunities and constraints of selected delivery media and the possible nature of student engagement. Factors such as time, costs, expertise, and infrastructure affect course design. The following steps are based on a traditional systems approach for designing distance education courses.

- Identify and divide course content into units or modules
- Identify available and required resources
- Decide on strategies for student assessment within each unit and throughout the course
- Design activities to engage students for each unit; decide which specific media will be used, and how these will influence production of the course
- Design the course template (Bates & Poole, 2003)

A less structured, more contemporary and constructivist approach is possible in distance courses. This does not suggest courses without boundaries, focus, or direction, but rather components that are more flexible and support student participation and control. Critical reflection, synthesis, evaluation of concepts and processes, and learning outcomes are achieved through

TABLE 9.4   CLASS GUIDELINES

Nursing 376 Teaching and Learning in Nursing Practice

Class Title: Course Synthesis

Overview

In this course you were invited to engage in various learning activities to build on and expand your knowledge in, and expertise with, teaching and learning interactions. Through our experiences, we addressed many of the foundational principles important in providing health education to clients and families. Now that the course is ending, it is important to reflect upon the growth achieved individually and collectively, recognize the new learning we have added to our teaching-learning repertoire, and critically evaluate the way(s) in which the knowledge and experiences in this course have influenced you as a learner and teacher.

Goals:

1. Reflect upon the course as a whole and critically evaluate how your knowledge and experiences about teaching and learning situations have been influenced.
2. Apply Bevis and Watson's interpretive-criticism model to appreciate both the obvious and the subtle learning achievements in this course.
3. Review the course and provide feedback to the professor.

In Preparation:

1. Examine the course as a whole and identify:
   a) insights that were new to you and made an impact upon you as a learner and as a professional
   b) areas in which you would like to pursue further professional development
2. Review course goals and identify strengths and limitations of the course in relation to achieving these goals individually and collectively.
3. Create a metaphor that symbolizes, and captures your experiences in this course.

In Class:

1. In small groups, discuss your perceptions, interpretations, and judgements about the course with classmates. Share key points with the class.
2. In small groups, discuss how your knowledge of critiquing can be applied to the group assignment completed in the course.
3. Offer constructive feedback about how the course might be further developed to support student learning.

On Reflection/Follow-up:

Reflect upon the insights you gained from your colleagues, readings, and experiences in this course. How will you continue to integrate your learning into your nursing practice?

learning activities. For example, sharing knowledge and experiences through dialogical learning, possible with asynchronous computer-conferencing, is compatible with a contemporary approach for distance delivery.

Teaching Strategies

Determining teaching strategies that enhance learning is an integral aspect of course design. Direct strategies, such as a lecture or small group discussion, require face-to-face interaction with students. The lecture may be complemented by indirect strategies such as readings from books and journals, or video-clips. When direct and indirect strategies are combined, they serve to stimulate learning through multiple sensory channels (VanHoozer et al., 1987).

Traditional Teaching Strategies Traditional teaching strategies are those that have been relied upon for decades, perhaps chosen by the instructor for convenience, comfort, and efficiency. The lecture, often selected as a primary classroom teaching strategy due to large class size, actively engages the instructor in the act of teaching. Students, however, may be more passively engaged in the learning process unless active learning strategies are incorporated into lectures (Oermann, 2004). Other examples of traditional strategies include discussions, seminars, questioning, and use of audio-visual equipment such as overheads or slides (DeYoung, 2003).

Contemporary Teaching Strategies Contemporary teaching strategies promote more active learner engagement than do traditional strategies. Students take an active role in learning experiences individually and/or with their colleagues through cooperative and collaborative projects, in computer-assisted instruction or other multimedia applications, and in virtual reality laboratories.

Clinical Teaching Strategies Teaching strategies for clinical courses are influenced by the setting, size, and level of the group, and the learning opportunities available. Pre- and post-conferences are commonly employed, as are direct client care and observational experiences, peer teaching, and preceptoring.

Distance Education Strategies Sound pedagogy is integral to all courses. In distance education, however, there is a risk that effective teaching could become secondary to the "bells and whistles" associated with the latest technologies. Careful planning is necessary to facilitate meaningful, substantive, and scholarly knowledge development in distance education. Teaching strategies should promote active learning in ways best suited to the technology. Student and educator preferences, as well as the time required to learn to use the technology, should be taken into account (Andrusyszyn, Cragg, & Humbert, 2001).

Much has been written about teaching strategies but it is beyond the scope of this text to examine each strategy in detail. Table 9.5 outlines characteristics that a novice nurse educa-

TABLE 9.5   CHARACTERISTICS OF COMMONLY USED TEACHING STRATEGIES

Teaching Strategy	Characteristics							
	Group Size	Cost	Infrastructure	Instructor Preparation Time	Learning Curve (Instructor)	Learner Engagement	Learning Curve (Student)	Intent
Algorithms	Both	Low	Low	High	Steep	Active	Minimal	Analysis, CT*
Audio-conferencing	Small	High	High	High	Moderate	Passive	Minimal	Understanding
Buzz Groups	Both	Low	Low	Low	Minimal	Active	Minimal	Application
Clinical Observation	Small	Low	Low	Medium	Minimal	Active	Moderate	Understanding
Computer-Assisted Instruction	Large	High	High	High	Steep	Active	Moderate	Application, Synthesis, CT
Computer-Conferencing	Small	High	High	High	Moderate	Active	Steep	Synthesis, Evaluation, CT
Concept mapping	Small	Low	Low	High	Moderate	Active	Moderate	Analysis, Synthesis, CT
Debate	Both	Low	Low	High	Steep	Active	Minimal	Analysis, CT
Direct Client Care	Small	Low	High	High	Steep	Active	Steep	Synthesis, Evaluation, CT
Gaming	Both	Low	Low	High	Moderate	Active	Minimal	Application, Synthesis, CT

continues

TABLE 9.5 CONTINUED

					Characteristics			
Teaching Strategy	Group Size	Cost	Infrastructure	Instructor Preparation Time	Learning Curve (Instructor)	Learner Engagement	Learning Curve (Student)	Intent
Laboratory Practice	Small	High	High	High	Moderate	Active	Moderate	Application, Synthesis, CT
Lecture	Large	Low	Low	High	Moderate	Passive	Minimal	Understanding
Lecture-Discussion	Large	Low	Low	High	Moderate	Active	Minimal	Understanding
Live Patient Simulations	Small	High	High	High	Steep	Active	Moderate	Application, Synthesis, CT
Metaphor	Both	Low	Low	High	Moderate	Active	Moderate	Critical reflection, Synthesis, CT
Multimedia	Large	High	High	High	Steep	Active	Steep	Application
Narrative Dialogue	Small	Low	Low	Medium	Moderate	Active	Minimal	Critical reflection, Synthesis, CT
One-Minute Paper	Both	Low	Low	Low	Minimal	Active	Minimal	Understanding
Oral Examinations	Small	Low	Low	High	Steep	Active	Steep	Evaluation, CT
Peer Teaching	Small	Low	Low	Medium	Moderate	Active	Steep	Understanding

Method								
Preceptorships	Small	Low	High	Medium	Low	Active	Minimal	Application, Synthesis, Evaluation, CT
Pre- and post-conferences	Small	Low	Low	High	Steep	Active	Minimal	Understanding, Synthesis, Evaluation, CT
Questioning	Both	Low	Low	High	Moderate	Active	Minimal	Understanding, Synthesis, Evaluation, CT
Reflective Journaling	Small	Low	Low	High	Moderate	Active	Steep	Critical reflection, Synthesis, CT
Role Play	Small	Low	Low	High	Moderate	Active	Moderate	Application, CT
Student Presentation	Both	Low	Low	High	Moderate	Active	Steep	Synthesis, CT
Think-Pair-Share	Large	High	Low	High	Minimal	Active	Minimal	Application, CT
Videoconferencing	Small	High	High	High	Steep	Active	Steep	Understanding, Synthesis
Videotape	Small	High	Low	High	Steep	Passive	Minimal	Understanding
Virtual Reality	Small	High	High	High	Steep	Active	Steep	Application, Synthesis, CT
Written Assignments	Both	Low	Low	High	Steep	Active	Moderate	Synthesis, Evaluation, CT

*CT = Critical Thinking

tor might find helpful when making decisions about using specific teaching strategies. In this Table, *group size* indicates the class size for which the strategy is suitable. *Cost and infrastructure* are the extent of financial and other organizational resources necessary to implement the strategy. *Instructor preparation time* refers to the amount of time required by an instructor to prepare a unit of learning using the specific strategy. *Learning curve* is a term adapted from industry that refers to the rate at which learning takes place to yield the desired outcome. If the learning curve associated with use of a specific teaching strategy is steep, then an alternate strategy may be considered. *Learner engagement* is the extent to which students participate in the learning process when a particular strategy is applied. *Intent* refers to the abilities expected of students.

Strategies to Evaluate Student Learning

Evaluation of student learning, a component of course design, requires thoughtful attention. Decisions about evaluation methods will be influenced by many factors, including: philosophical approaches, course goals, purpose of the evaluation (formative/summative), content, course level, learning domain, class size, educational delivery medium, reliability, validity, utility, evaluation frequency, and availability of resources to implement the preferred strategies.

A wide range of strategies can be used to assess student learning in classroom and clinical courses, either individually or in combination. As well, consideration should be given to whether students have evaluation options or can propose their own assignments. Strategies are not described here in detail; however, more commonly used evaluation approaches include:

- portfolios, simulation, role play, critiquing, journal-writing, scholarly papers, essays, verbal questioning, concept or mind mapping, audiotape, and videotape (Kirkpatrick, DeWitt-Weaver, & Yeager, 1998)
- oral reports and articles for publication (de Tornyay & Thompson, 1987)
- checklists, rating scales, anecdotal reports (Van Hoozer, et al., 1987)
- observation, process recordings, care plans, teaching plans, clinical documentation (Reilly & Oermann, 1999)
- written and clinical performance examinations, self-reports, and peer evaluation

Course Design Process

Designing a course is an iterative process with decisions about each course component affecting decisions about other components. The process involves writing, modifying, critiquing, and revising before plans are finalized. The intent is to devise a course that adheres to curriculum philosophical approaches, facilitates students' achievement of curriculum goals, and is effective within the school's context. There should be unity within the course, such that the relationships among the course components are apparent.

Course titles, brief descriptions, placement in the program, general goals, predominant concepts, etc. are determined as part of the process of curriculum design (see Chapter 8). These, along with ideas about curriculum possibilities (content and learning experiences) generated during analysis of contextual data (see Chapter 6), are reviewed as intensive course design begins.

Typically, courses are designed in the order in which they are to be implemented. During the design process, courses should be compared to the curriculum matrix (if one exists) to maintain adherence to the original curriculum intent. Reasons for deviations should be explained and agreement reached about their acceptability. Variations from the curriculum matrix might necessitate changes in subsequent courses (Heinrich, Karner, Gaglione, & Lambert, 2002).

Course design is not an activity undertaken in isolation. Ongoing consultation is required among course designers to ensure that the curriculum intent and integrity are maintained, concurrent courses are complementary, sequenced courses build in depth and complexity without redundancy, curriculum goals can be achieved, and student workload is reasonable.

As described below, the design process begins with a review of parameters and a choice of course design approach, and then proceeds to creation of the course components. Although attention is given to the components individually, ideas arise about all of them simultaneously. This concurrent thinking promotes course unity. The process concludes with a critique of the course design and preparation of information for students.

Reviewing Course Parameters

Course design begins with a firm understanding of the course parameters. To crystallize the parameters in the minds of those designing courses, faculty might ask:

- What are the institutional requirements related to course design?
- What are the implications of the philosophical approaches for course design?
- What is the learning climate we wish to achieve in the course?
- What is the structure for this course?
- Which delivery method(s) will be employed? Could multiple methods be used? Is the infrastructure available to support the preferred method(s)?
- What resources will be available for the course?
- What is the class size?
- What are the knowledge and experiences that students bring to this course?

- What are the students' characteristics?
- Will the students be:
  - direct from secondary institutions?
  - those with previous diplomas, degrees, or some post-secondary education?
  - adults with strong values about lifelong learning who are continuing their education?
  - individuals who, in addition to academic responsibilities, juggle multiple life roles?
  - learners with special needs for whom certain accommodations need to be made?
  - diverse or homogenous?

Choosing an Approach for Course Design

The choice of an approach for course design could be guided by the following questions:

- Will a traditional, contemporary, or blended approach best fit with the philosophical approaches of the curriculum?
- Which approach is consistent with faculty and student preferences?
- Which approach is practical in our situation?
- Are there institutional requirements that influence our choice?

Identifying the Course Purpose and Description

Identifying the course purpose sets the stage for subsequent discussion. Course designers should consider:

- What is the reason this course is in the curriculum?
- What is the main intent of this course?
- How does this course move students toward semester and curriculum goals?

A preliminary course description is written, and this undergoes many revisions during course design. The initial description represents the ideas that faculty first discuss as possibilities for the course. The course description is not finalized until all other components of course design are completed. In general, the following questions are raised as the description is discussed and written.

- What should this course be about?
- When could it best be offered (days, evenings, weekends)?
- What kinds of learning experiences could occur in the course?

- What would be the nature of interactions in these learning experiences?
- What could be the scope of the content, or the nature of practice experiences?
- How would we like students to participate in this course?

Formulating Course Goals

The general course goals developed during the curriculum design process are refined, and perhaps expanded, to more closely reflect the emerging design. Semester goals are analyzed to identify the competencies and then course goals are written to include concepts and context particular to that course. Formulation of course goals centers on the queries listed below.

- Which of the semester goals could this course address?
- Which aspects of the semester goals seem most suitable for this course?
- What concepts and processes should course goals reflect?
- What is the context in which goal achievement will be demonstrated?

Determining Content

Educators might pose the following questions when selecting content for each course.

- What is important content for this course?
- What portions of the possible content will contribute most meaningfully to students' achievements of learning goals?
- What is a reasonable depth and scope of content at this stage of the nursing curriculum?
- What content can best illustrate the concepts to be addressed in the course?
- How can the content be organized and sequenced to emphasize philosophical approaches and curriculum goals?

Deciding on Classes

The division of the content into conceptually meaningful and logically sequenced units comprises the creation of classes. Course designers could consider:

- How many class sessions will there be?
- How can the content be grouped so it is meaningful and logical, and so that it matches the number of class sessions?
- What goals should be emphasized through which content?

- If titles are assigned to each class, what will they be? Do these titles reflect the philosophical approaches and nature of the content?

Selecting Teaching Strategies

Selection of teaching strategies is of vital concern to course designers since these define, in part, what faculty will do. As course faculty members ponder the wide range of strategies and techniques available to them, they give thought to the following questions.

- What strategies best align with our philosophical approaches?
- Which are congruent with curriculum goals?
- Which are feasible within the course parameters?
- Which are suitable for our delivery method(s)?
- Which best suit students' learning needs and styles?
- Which are compatible with faculty teaching styles and preferences?

Creating Student Learning Activities

Formulating student learning activities calls upon the creativity of course designers. Questions they might ask include:

- What types of student engagement with content will promote achievement of course goals?
- What activities can facilitate students' achievement of course goals?
- What readings and other resources will enhance student learning?
- If distance education is used, which learning activities are compatible with the delivery medium proposed? What issues might be anticipated in relation to the medium?

Planning for Evaluation of Student Learning

Decisions about the types of evaluation methods, nature and frequency of evaluation, student choices among methods, and the provision of criteria to students, are among the decisions that faculty make when designing courses. Among the questions to be considered are:

- Which evaluation methods would best assess students' achievement of course goals?
- What types of evaluation procedures will be congruent with the curriculum philosophical approaches?
- What are the advantages and disadvantages of the preferred strategies?
- How and when might formative and summative evaluation approaches be used?

- How will evaluation components be weighted? Will students have the option of determining their own weightings?
- Should there be options for student selection of evaluation methods? If so, how can we plan this?
- Will student self-evaluation be included?

Critiquing Course Design

As course design proceeds, faculty engage in ongoing appraisal. Before finalizing the course design they critique it in a more holistic fashion, asking themselves:

- Is this course feasible within the design parameters?
- Is it reasonable within the faculty workload?
- Is the course congruent with the curriculum philosophical approaches?
- Is the course likely to lead to students' achievement of course goals?
- Is the course design reasonable in view of requirements that students must meet for other courses in the semester?
- Do written descriptions of course components reflect our intent in a way that will be meaningful to others?
- Have we taken student diversity into account?

Preparing Course Packages

Once decisions have been made about the course design, a course package, or syllabus, can be prepared for students. This compendium could be available for purchase by students or posted on a course web site. The terminology and precise nature of the packages vary depending on faculty values. The following might be included: an expanded course description; course goals; evaluation methods; schedule, topics, and student guidelines for course sessions. As well, a compilation of journal articles and other materials can be prepared. While a reading package is convenient for students, faculty must assemble it early enough for copyright permission to be obtained and for reproduction. Internet access to journal articles can minimize the size of this package and facilitate student retrieval.

Designing Individual Classes

The overall course design provides the framework for individual classes. Each class must contribute to the course purpose, with student learning activities particularized for each class. When planning classes, teachers might ask:

- How can the class be designed to clearly relate to course goals?
- What should students achieve in this class?
- What should happen so that the class purpose is achieved? What should the students be doing? What should the teacher be doing?
- What is a reasonable sequence and time allotment for the activities?

If a traditional approach to course design is employed, lesson plans (Table 9.3) can be developed to organize each class. If a blended approach is used, class guidelines developed for students can be beneficial. With either approach, class planning generally involves determining the:

- purpose or goals students should achieve
- scope of content
- teaching strategies
- learning activities to engage students
- sequence and timing of class activities

Within each class, there are a number of instructional events that teachers should arrange, according to Gagné, Briggs, and Wager (1992). Although the events are described in a behaviorist fashion, they have relevance for most classes. Table 9.6 lists the nine events and provides examples of how they could be enacted. It is important to note that one teaching activity can simultaneously encompass more than one instructional event. For example, questioning can be used to both elicit and assess performance. An understanding of these instructional events can help teachers plan classes in which student participation is required, learning is assessed, and transfer of learning is taken into account.

Many teachers like to obtain feedback about each class. Therefore, they plan a few minutes at the conclusion of each session to ask students questions such as:

- What did you like about this class?
- What worked well for you?
- What might we have done differently?

This information allows for refinement of the class if it is to be conducted in subsequent semesters. As well, if a pattern of response emerges in reaction to the predominant teaching strategies, it is possible to take this into account for subsequent classes.

Faculty Development

Faculty development for course design is directed towards facilitating members' knowledge and expertise in designing courses. Depending on faculty needs, and following an ini-

TABLE 9.6   EXAMPLES OF TEACHER ACTIVITIES FOR INSTRUCTIONAL EVENTS

Instructional Events	Examples of Teacher Activities
Gaining attention	State the focus of the class
	Provide or ask for a clinical example
Informing learner of objectives	Describe the purpose of the class
	State class goals
Stimulating recall of prerequisite knowledge	Ask for significant points from previous class or required reading
	Ask how required reading for present class relates to previous learning
Presenting the stimulus material	Lecture with audio-video augmentation
	Ask questions to initiate and stimulate group discussion
	Ask students to role-play
	Have students debate
	Have students do class presentation
	Use narrative dialogue
Providing learning guidance	Provide hints, non-verbal cues
	Ask additional questions
Eliciting student performance	Ask questions
	Pose problems
	Present cases for analysis
Providing feedback about performance correctness	Confirm responses
	Rephrase or redirect question
Assessing the performance	Ask questions
	Gauge quality of discussion
	Use directed paraphrasing
Enhancing retention and transfer	Summarize and synthesize
	Ask students for summary and synthesis
	Ask how understandings will influence practice
	Ask for one-minute papers

[Some data from Gagné, R.M., Briggs, L.J., & Wager, W.W. (1992). *Principles of instructional design.* (4th ed.). Fort Worth: Harcourt, Brace, Jovanovich College Publishers].

tial review session on the parameters involved, faculty development activities can include discussion about some or all of the course components.

Discussion about the approach to course design would be appropriate. This would help team members appreciate whether a traditional, contemporary, blended, or distance approach would be most relevant to the curriculum's philosophical base and goals. Mentorship to help those less familiar with course and class design could be beneficial. Course designers might also gain from microteaching sessions to practice new teaching strategies proposed for courses. This could be followed by member critiques.

Likely, some attention will have to be given to drafting course and class designs. This may be a first activity for some. Sharing, critiquing, and discussing can be facilitated by experienced members.

Chapter Summary

In this chapter, course components, that is, the description, purpose, goals, teaching strategies, content, classes, student learning activities, and evaluation of learning are described. The parameters that influence course design are detailed. Several approaches to course design are described, including distance education. Teaching and evaluation strategies are overviewed. Attention is given to the process of course design and ideas are presented for the design of individual classes. The intent is that courses reflect the philosophical approaches and are structured to facilitate student achievement of course goals and, ultimately, semester and curriculum goals. Activities for faculty development are offered.

Synthesis Activities

Two case studies are presented below. The Senyk University case is followed by a critique. Discuss the case and its analysis, considering additional ideas that arise. The second, Philmore University, is followed by questions to guide examination of the case. Curriculum development activities are proposed for consideration in individual settings.

Senyk University

Senyk University School of Nursing has been offering RN-BSN education for fifteen years. Normally there are approximately 40 students in attendance at classes. The approach most often used is small group discussions about nursing course content in rooms with moveable tables and chairs.

Faculty realize that their students are adult learners with multiple roles, and that attendance at on-campus classes is a challenge for some. Most students are from neighboring towns, although a few are from more distant areas. For many years, students have asked for courses to be accessible by distance education.

Two of the nine faculty members, Rachel and Naomi, have been integrating more technology into their courses. They have posted their course outlines on websites and used chat rooms to respond to occasional course-related questions. Rachel and Naomi have asked the Dean for permission to mount their courses entirely through video-conferencing. They view this as an opportunity to pilot these courses in the next semester and then evaluate the outcomes. Senyk University has state-of-the-art video-conferencing suites, and infrastructure to support web-based course delivery that includes conferencing. Rachel and Naomi are confident that the courses will be well received by students.

Critique It is commendable that faculty at Senyk University are interested in re-designing their courses for distance delivery. The time they have to make necessary design changes is of concern. It would be valuable for them to discuss instructional design relevant to their course goals with consultants in the university educational development office. Exploring the features of the available media, and their congruence with course goals, will inform them about possibilities they may not have considered. Faculty in other divisions may also be helpful as mentors during this process.

In their eagerness to meet students' requests, the faculty have not adequately considered how video-conferencing would suit their intentions. Although video-conferencing facilities are available on campus, this medium is time- and place-dependent, and it is not clear if out-of-town students can access similar technology. As well, video-conferencing does not allow the flexibility possible with other time- and place-independent technologies. While small group discussions in face-to-face classes are reasonable, a video-conferencing design will require exceptional organizational skills to keep groups focused and allow time for synthesis and shared learning from all groups. Moreover, the costs have not been considered.

Faculty might explore how existing web-based computer conferencing can be used for their courses. Asynchronous and periodic synchronous discussions organized online could promote integrative learning and allow for shared decision-making. If appropriate, video-conferencing could be scheduled periodically throughout the term, for example, when guest lectures are included, or for synthesis activities. In such a course, a print package of information and course materials could be sent to students or posted on the web before the course begins. This would help students prepare for and begin the course.

Philmore College

Situated in a small, non-industrial town, Philmore College was originally a "hilltop" college established in 1818 as a school for boys and later, for boys and girls. The school has evolved into a 4-year, privately endowed, non-sectarian, post-secondary institution. Since the 1960's, programs leading to baccalaureate degrees in psychosocial and physical sciences have been offered. An 18-month accelerated program in baccalaureate nursing education was inaugurated in 1996 for applicants with a prior degree. The purpose of the program was to graduate more BSN nurses in a shorter period of time in response to the shortage of nurses.

The 11 master's-prepared full-time nursing faculty have combined nursing practice and teaching experience ranging from 4–18 years. The director, Agnes Philmore, a direct descendant of the founder, joined Philmore College in 1996, and is currently pursuing doctoral studies by distance education. All nursing faculty, including the director, engage in classroom and clinical teaching. The practice experiences are offered in one local 200-bed community hospital, a 224-bed tertiary care hospital in a neighboring city, and a 76-bed long-term and residential care facility. Students also have community nursing experience, which is coordinated and supervised by a primary care nurse practitioner with an adjunct faculty appointment.

The Philmore nursing education program is discipline-specific. Credit for non-nursing support and elective courses is given automatically to students who qualify for admission. Approximately 85 students graduate annually and have been consistently successful in the licensure examinations and in obtaining employment.

The director, faculty, several students, and the nurse practitioner, who comprise the curriculum committee, have held several meetings over the past four months to revamp the curriculum. A review of the parameters has been completed, and a change from their traditional philosophy to a feminist-humanist philosophical approach has been articulated. The curriculum goals have been rewritten to more clearly reflect the unique characteristics of the graduates and their role as professionals. As agreed, the accelerated 18-month program will continue to be discipline-specific, and the committee is ready to begin course design.

Agnes Philmore scheduled a workshop for the curriculum committee to consider a more contemporary course design approach. The tasks now are to determine the course design approach and then to design the courses.

Questions for Consideration and Analysis of the Philmore College Case

1. What parameters must the curriculum committee consider when designing the courses?
2. In what way will the feminist-humanist perspective influence course design?
3. What components should be included in the courses?
4. What classroom and clinical experiences could be incorporated in the courses?
5. What teaching and learning approaches would be appropriate for the courses?
6. Design a sample course for this accelerated baccalaureate-nursing program.

Curriculum Development Activities for Consideration in Your Setting

Use the following questions to guide thinking about your course design.

1. How will the parameters influence our decisions about course design?

2. Which approach(es) to course design will we choose, and why?

3. What should be the purpose, description, and goals of the courses?

4. What is the scope of content for the courses?

5. What learning activities should we consider to facilitate students' achievement of course goals?

6. Which teaching strategies could be used?

7. Which evaluation approaches should we consider?

8. What are faculty learning needs related to course design?

References

Andrusyszyn, M.A.(1998). Instructor's Guide to Computer Conferencing. Retrieved March 13, 2004, from http://publish.uwo.ca/~maandrus/cmcgui~1.htm

Andrusyszyn, M.A., Cragg, B., & Humbert, J. (2001). Nurse practitioner preferences for distance education methods related to learning style, course content, and achievement. *The Journal of Nursing Education, 40*(4), 1–8.

Bates, A., & Poole, G. (2003). Effective teaching with technology in higher education: Foundations for success. San Francisco, CA.: Jossey-Bass.

Bevis, E.O. (1982). *Curriculum building in nursing: A process.* (3rd ed.). St. Louis: C.V. Mosby Company.

Bevis, E.O. (2000a). Nursing education as professional education: some underlying theoretical issues. In E.O. Bevis & J. Watson (Eds.), *Toward a caring curriculum. A new pedagogy for nursing.* (pp. 67–106). Boston: Jones and Bartlett Publishers.

Bevis, E.O. (2000b). Teaching and learning. The key to education and professionalism. In E.O. Bevis & J. Watson (Eds.), *Toward a caring curriculum. A new pedagogy for nursing.* (pp. 153–188). Boston: Jones and Bartlett Publishers.

Bowe, F.G. (2000). *Universal Design in Education: Teaching Nontraditional Students.* Westport, CT: Bergin & Garvey.

de Tornyay, R. & Thompson, M. (1987). *Strategies for teaching nursing.* (3rd ed.). New York: Wiley.

DeYoung, S. (2003). *Teaching strategies for nurse educators.* Upper Saddle River, New Jersey: Prentice Hall.

Diekelmann, D. (2001). Narrative pedagogy: Heideggerian hermeneutical analyses of lived experiences of students, teachers, and clinicians. *Advances in Nursing Science, 23*(3), 53–71.

Gagné, R.M., Briggs, L.J., & Wager, W.W. (1992). Principles of instructional design. (4th ed.). Fort Worth, PA: Harcourt, Brace, Jovanovich College Publishers.

Goldenberg, D. & Iwasiw, C.L. (1992). Reciprocal learning among students in the clinical areas. *Nurse Educator, 17*(5), 27–29.

Heinrich, C.R., Karner, K.J., Gaglione, B.H., & Lambert, L.S. (2002). Order out of chaos. The use of a matrix to validate curriculum integrity. *Nurse Educator, 27*(3), 136–140.

Ironside, P.M. (2003). New pedagogies for teaching thinking: The lived experiences of students and teachers enacting narrative pedagogy. *Journal of Nursing Education,* 42, 509–513.

Ironside, P.M. (2004). "Covering content" and teaching thinking: Deconstructing the additive curriculum. *Journal of Nursing Education, 43*(1), 5–12.

Iwasiw, C.L. (1987). The role of teacher in self-directed learning. *Nurse Education Today, 7,* 222–227.

Iwasiw, C.L. & Goldenberg, D. (1993). Peer teaching among students in the clinical area: Effects on student learning. *Journal of Advanced Nursing, 18,* 659–668.

Kirkpatrick, J.M., DeWitt-Weaver, D., & and Yeager, L. (1998). Strategies for evaluating learning outcomes. In D.M. Billings & J.A. Halstead (Eds.), *Teaching in nursing: A guide for faculty.* (pp. 367–384). Philadelphia: W.B. Saunders Company.

Oermann, M.H. (2004). Using active learning in lectures: Best of "both worlds". *International Journal of Nursing Education Scholarship, 1.* Retrieved February 28, 2004, from http://www.bepress.com/injes/vol1/iss1/art1/

Reilly, D.E. & Oermann, M.H. (1999). *Clinical Teaching in Nursing Education.* (2nd ed.). Boston: Jones and Bartlett Publishers.

Saunders, S. & Kardia, D. (n.d.). Creating inclusive college classrooms. Center for Research on Learning and Teaching, University of Michigan. Retrieved April 21, 2004, from http://www.crlt.umich.edu/gsis/P3_1.html

Seaton-Sykes, P. (2003). Teaching and learning in Internet environment in Australian nursing education. Unpublished doctoral dissertation. Griffith University, Queensland, Australia.

Van Hoozer, H.L., Bratton, B.D., Ostmoe, P.M., Weinholtz, D., Craft, M.J., Gjerde, C.L., & Albanese, M.A. (1987). *The teaching process: Theory and practice in nursing.* Norwalk, Connecticut: Appleton-Century-Crofts.

Watson, J. (2000). A new paradigm of curriculum development. In E.O. & J. Watson (Eds.), *Toward a caring curriculum. A new pedagogy for nursing.* (pg. 37). Boston: Jones and Bartlett Publishers.

CHAPTER 10

Planning Curriculum Evaluation

Chapter Overview

Planning for curriculum evaluation is an ongoing process, which begins simultaneously with curriculum design. Nursing faculty and administrators are responsible for appraising the overall curriculum. The definition, purposes, and models of curriculum evaluation are described. Planning for evaluation, establishing standards, and determining data collection approaches are addressed. Contained also is more specific information about planning for the evaluation of curriculum goals, design, and outcomes; courses; teaching and evaluation strategies; human and physical resources; learning climate; and policies. A brief discussion of faculty development activities related to planning for curriculum evaluation is followed by the chapter summary, and synthesis activities. These include two cases for discussion, and questions to guide evaluation planning in individual settings.

Chapter Goals

- Appreciate evaluation planning as a component of curriculum development
- Understand the purposes of curriculum evaluation
- Gain insight into models of curriculum evaluation

- Consider evaluation of individual curriculum components
- Recognize the value of faculty development for curriculum development

Definition and Purposes of Curriculum Evaluation

Definition of Curriculum Evaluation

Curriculum evaluation is an organized and thoughtful appraisal of those elements central to the course of studies undertaken by students, as well as of the abilities of those students as graduates. It involves establishing standards for judging quality, systematic data collection, application of the standards, and formulation of judgments about the value, quality, utility, effectiveness or significance (Fitzpatrick, Sanders, & Worthen, 2004) of the curriculum. The aspects to be evaluated include the curriculum goals, design, and outcomes; courses; teaching and evaluation strategies; human and physical resources to support the curriculum; learning climate; and curriculum policies.

In contrast, *program evaluation* encompasses a wider scope of elements to be assessed. In addition to all aspects of curriculum evaluation, program evaluation includes attention to institutional support for the school; administrative structure of the school; faculty members' teaching, research, and professional activities; the school's relationships with other academic units; and student support services.

Purposes of Internal Curriculum Evaluation

Internal curriculum evaluation is conducted by members of the school to determine the strengths and weaknesses of the curriculum. It is undertaken to establish student achievement of the curriculum goals, and to monitor students' learning experiences while in the program (Pateman & Jinks, 1999), thereby providing a basis for review, modification, and reorganization of the curriculum. Essentially, it is a quality control mechanism to assure that the curriculum, its courses, the processes undertaken, teaching strategies, and student achievement of goals are meeting the required standards. Curriculum evaluation can provide justification for refinement, revision, or complete curriculum change.

Formative evaluation is carried out at regular intervals during the implementation of a new curriculum. The purpose is to provide evidence about the feasibility and effectiveness of a portion of the curriculum, so that ongoing revisions and improvements can be made. Evidence comes mainly from teachers and students.

Summative evaluation is carried out at the completion of a portion of, or the total curriculum. The purpose is to judge the effectiveness of all or part of the curriculum. Evidence comes from teachers, students, graduates, administrators, and other stakeholders. Summative evaluation is also performed to compare one curriculum with another (Ediger, Snyder, &

Corcoran, 1983; Gagné, Briggs & Wager, 1992). Both formative and summative evaluations address curriculum effectiveness and assist in decision-making about curriculum.

Purposes of External Curriculum Evaluation

Curriculum evaluation is undertaken as part of a more extensive program evaluation conducted for approval or accreditation by an external agency. State or provincial approval and national accreditation are processes by which an external organization evaluates and recognizes an institution or program of study as meeting certain predetermined criteria.

Approval Nursing program approval is a compulsory evaluation or review process concerned primarily with the protection of public interests. Approval indicates that a nursing program is of a quality sufficient for graduates to be allowed to write the licensing examination. Protection of public interests is accomplished by ensuring that a program has met prescribed minimum standards set by a body designated in state or provincial legislation, or according to regulations authorized by that legislation. Every nursing program leading to licensure examinations must meet the standards of the body authorized to regulate nursing. The schools cannot operate without approval, since graduates would not be eligible to write the licensing examination.

In the United States, approval by state Boards of Nursing is required for all nursing education programs. In Canada, approval is granted by provincial nursing associations or by a provincial College of Nurses, except for Ontario baccalaureate programs. The Ontario College of Nurses requires that all baccalaureate programs have national accreditation.

Accreditation Accreditation is an endorsement of a nursing program by a nongovernmental agency concerned with nursing education; national accreditation is understood to connote excellence. The accreditation process is voluntary (except for baccalaureate programs in Ontario), and is a rigorous appraisal of the curriculum and other aspects of the program. Accreditation standards are set by the profession. The degree to which a program or institution conforms to these standards is determined through the accreditation process (Joel, 2003). Accreditation can be important in attracting students and faculty, and can influence a school's eligibility for outside funding, graduates' entrance to subsequent programs, and students' ability to obtain grants or loans.

The major accrediting organization for licensed practical, diploma, and associate degree nursing programs in the United States is the National League for Nursing Accrediting Commission (NLNAC). Baccalaureate and graduate nursing programs are accredited by the NLNAC and the Commission on Collegiate Nursing Education. In Canada, accreditation exists only for baccalaureate programs. The Canadian Association of Schools of Nursing (CASN) is the accrediting body.

There are many purposes of curriculum evaluation, all of which are related, and none of which is mutually exclusive. The purposes are listed in Table 10.1.

TABLE 10.1   PURPOSES OF CURRICULUM EVALUATION

1. Diagnose curriculum problems; assess strengths and weaknesses.
2. Examine intended and actual effects of the curriculum.
3. Document achievement of the curriculum in relation to the learning goals.
4. Determine if the curriculum is effective.
5. Provide data to make curriculum and administrative decisions.
6. Assist the dean or director and faculty to account for fiscal resources.
7. Apprise dean or director of faculty development needs.
8. Fulfill approval and/or accreditation requirements.

Curriculum Evaluation Models

A curriculum evaluation model is a framework that guides the evaluation of a curriculum. Variations in models arise from differing conceptions and definitions of *evaluation*. Accordingly, they differ in the emphasis placed on the curriculum aspects to be examined, the approaches to data collection, and the basis of judging the quality of the curriculum. The models provide a path for planning and conducting evaluation, not a detailed roadmap.

Evaluation models and approaches range from checklists and suggestions to comprehensive appraisals. In nursing education, evaluation of the total curriculum is comprehensive. It is typically based on standards of quality and incorporates both quantitative and qualitative approaches.

Quantitative models, e.g., Scriven's goal-free model and Provus' discrepancy model, incorporate predetermined criteria and structure. In contrast, qualitative models are more open. For example, Guba's naturalistic model addresses the concerns, claims, and issues of stakeholders, and the methods to examine these are negotiated with stakeholders. In qualitative approaches, data are obtained through direct observations and interviews rather than questionnaires as is typical in quantitative approaches (Chavesse, 1994).

Each evaluation approach has particular strengths that can help illuminate different aspects of the curriculum. Therefore, selection of a curriculum evaluation model, or evaluation approach, should be contingent upon the purpose of the evaluation, the questions to be addressed, the issues that must be taken into account, available resources, and any faculty preference for one model over another. Applegate (1998) suggests the chosen model should be based "on the faculty's beliefs about education [and] the political and institutional context in which the program exists" (p. 183).

Whichever model(s) can provide the best evidence to answer the questions within the resource constraints would be a good choice. It is also possible to use a combination of relevant concepts from different models. This eclectic approach, while not an evaluation model as such, might offer more scope than one model, as well as mature, diverse, and sophisticated evaluation strategies (Fitzpatrick et al., 2004).

Typology of Evaluation Models

Models of evaluation have been categorized into many typologies. Each classification system presents a different perspective on educational and service program evaluation, even though many of the same models are included. For example, Stufflebeam, Madaus, and Kellaghan (2000) categorized models as questions/methods-oriented, improvement/accountability-oriented, and social agenda (advocacy)-oriented. Fitzpatrick et al. (2004) categorize them as: objectives-, management-, consumer-, expertise-, and participant-oriented. Guba and Lincoln's (1989) typology classifies models according to first, second, third and fourth generations, according to the evaluation focus. See Table 10.2 for a summary of the four generations of evaluation models.

Many curriculum and program evaluation models used in nursing education and service are third generation models. Several are summarized in Table 10.3. Increasingly, however, third and fourth generation models are combined to yield richer evaluations.

Planning Curriculum Evaluation

Planning curriculum evaluation is a dimension of curriculum development that should occur simultaneously with curriculum and course design. It is prudent to remember that curriculum evaluation is only one aspect of a school's activities and, therefore, the undertaking must be confined to what is necessary to achieve the purposes of the evaluation. Decisions are made about the:

- selection of an evaluation model
- relevant data
- methods and timing of data collection
- individuals who will interpret and judge the evidence
- purposes to be achieved by curriculum evaluation (why and for whom it is necessary)
- individual or committee responsible for overseeing the curriculum evaluation

TABLE 10.2   SUMMARY OF FIRST, SECOND, THIRD, AND FOURTH GENERATION EVALUATION MODELS

First Generation (technical)	**Measurement** (Prior to WW1): Students were targeted for evaluation. Tests were developed to measure variables of interest. Student scores were used to determine curriculum success.
Second Generation (description and technical)	**Description** (Post WW1): Curriculum was targeted for evaluation in an objectives-oriented (Tylerian) description approach (patterns, strengths, and weaknesses related to specific objectives). Congruence between student performance and described objectives was assessed. The program, materials, teaching strategies, organizational patterns, and "treatments" were evaluated. Measurement was redefined as one of several tools to use.
Third Generation (judgment-based, description, and technical)	**Judgment** (Post 1967): Program goals and performance were targeted for evaluation. Judgments about merit and worth were based on standards. Information collected depended on the evaluation model, e.g., decisions (decision-oriented models); experienced "effects" (goal-free models); internalized guideposts (connoisseurship models).
Fourth Generation (holistic and inclusive)	**Responsive, Constructivist, Naturalistic** (Post late 1970s): Took into account the claims (values), concerns, and issues of those involved in the evaluation (students, faculty, clients, administrators). It is a *responsive* (determines parameters and boundaries through an interactive, negotiated process that involves stakeholders), *constructivist* (interpretive, hermeneutic, relates to the methodology employed), *naturalistic,* (rejects the controlling, manipulative, experimental approach), sociopolitical, diagnostic, change-oriented, educative process. Results in a constructed understanding of needed improvements and changes, based on consensus of all stakeholders.

(Some data from Guba, E., & Lincoln, Y. (1989). *Fourth Generation Evaluation.* Newbury Park, CA: Sage.)

Resolution of these matters in advance of curriculum implementation will allow for organized formative and summative evaluation. The ongoing accumulation of data, which will contribute meaningfully to subsequent external reviews, provides evidence of a commitment to continuous curriculum improvement. Attention to the elements of systematic program evaluation (NLNAC, 2003) can guide faculty in the development of a curriculum evaluation plan.

TABLE 10.3   SUMMARY OF SEVERAL THIRD GENERATION EVALUATION MODELS

Model	Description
Scriven's (1967, 1972) goal-free	Measures all outcomes/effects of program, regardless of program goals or objectives. There are no pre-specified objectives. May be applied to total or sections of the curriculum.
Donabedian's (1969) quality assurance	Measures efficiency and effectiveness of courses or units of study. Component parts include trial, structure, purpose, and output.
Stufflebeam's (1971) CIPP	Involves decisions about planning (Context); structuring (Input); implementing (Process); and recycling (Product). Investigates students' needs and problems. A quality control, monitoring system that measures finances, personnel, facilities, and program effectiveness.
Provus' (1971) discrepancy evaluation	Compares performance with standards to determine if a discrepancy exists between the two. Includes 5 stages: definition of program, installation of program, process, product or outcomes, and cost-benefit analysis. Involves intended vs. actual outcomes, and effects.
Stake's (1972) (countenance) congruence-contingency	Involves congruence (agreement between desired and actual outcomes), and contingency (relationship among variables). Takes into account: *antecedents* (characteristics of students, teachers, curriculum, facilities, materials, organization, community); *transactions* (all educational experiences); *outcomes* (abilities, achievements, and attitudes resulting from educational experience).
Renzulli's (1972) key features	Considers major concerns of groups who have a direct or indirect interest in the program. Key features are prime interest groups and time.
Parlett & Hamilton's (1972) illuminative evaluation	Proposes that understanding of the curriculum is possible only in its wider contexts and in the biography of each course. The approach is not pre-determined but develops as issues or problems are identified. It is an ethno-graphic approach with two core concepts: instructional systems (courses) and learning milieu.

continues

TABLE 10.3   CONTINUED

Model	Description
Stenhouse (1975)	Discloses meaning of curriculum, purposes of courses, problems amenable to solutions, influence of context on curriculum, and whether the evaluation contributes to theory development. Includes five criteria: meaning, potential, interest, conditionality, and elucidation.
Starpoli and Waltz (1978)	Includes specific questions of concern to varied audiences, depending on what is being evaluated. Specifies decision-makers for each question, i.e., who should be responsible for evaluation activities, and how evaluation will proceed. There are four distinct, interrelated levels of evaluation: school, program, subprogram, course level; and three frames: input, operations, output.
Eisner's (1977, 1985) connoisseur/ critic	Premise is that experts (connoisseurs) can understand and appreciate subtle qualities of the classroom or program, and merits of the teacher and curriculum.
Stufflebeam's (1983) educational decision	Educational decision-making model that addresses four concerns: a) *context*: setting, mission, community, philosophy, internal/external focus; b) *input*: resources, support systems; learners, program plan; c) *process*: implementation, teaching/learning strategies and transactions, learning materials, efficiency and effectiveness; d) *product*: learner outcomes and satisfaction; all to facilitate decision-making.
Stake's (1991) education	Is organized around issues and concerns of stakeholders (students, faculty, administrators, parents, employers); goal is to discover merits and weakness of the program. Uses methods to generate data responsive to identified issues and concerns.

[Some data from Herbener, D.J., & Watson, J.E. (1992). Evaluating nursing education programs. *Nursing Outlook, 40* (1), 28; Stufflebeam, D.L., Madaus, G.F., & Kellaghan, T. (Eds.). (2000). *Evaluation models. Viewpoints on educational and human services evaluation*. (2nd ed.). Boston: Kluwer Academic Publishers.]

Decisions made when planning curriculum evaluation are not made separately. Rather, they are based on discussions that arise from the following questions:

- What are faculty's beliefs and values about curriculum evaluation?
- What is the purpose of the evaluation?

- Which evaluation model(s) are congruent with the curriculum?
- What will constitute quality?
- How often and when should the curriculum be evaluated?
- What aspects of the curriculum should be evaluated?
- Which sources can provide information needed for evaluation?
- Which established data-collection tools could be used? Are they appropriate?
- If school-specific instruments are needed, who will design them?
- How can data be organized and interpreted to arrive at important curricular evaluation conclusions?
- How will evaluation results be used?
- Who will be responsible for managing the evaluation process?

Generally, curriculum evaluation activities are shared among all faculty. Yet, the overall responsibility must rest with an individual or group, such as the curriculum committee, so that the efforts are coordinated and complete. Documenting the evaluation efforts and recording evaluation results and subsequent curriculum changes will provide information important for internal and external evaluation. Moreover, evidence of systematic and ongoing evaluation, and the results of these appraisals, are required for accreditation.

Establishing Standards, Criteria, and Indicators

Decisions about curriculum effectiveness and quality depend on a clear understanding of the standards against which the curriculum is being judged and the criteria whose achievement show that the standards are being attained. Standards are the "agreed upon rules to measure quantity, extent, value, and quality. Criteria are statements which identify the variables that need to be examined in evaluation of a standard" (NLNAC, 2003, p.12).

Delineation of precise criteria for all curriculum components is not possible. Therefore, formulating the indicators that point to achievement of the standards may be appropriate. As well, agreement must be reached about whether the standards are absolute or relative (Fitzpatrick et al., 2004). The specification of standards, criteria, and indicators allows faculty to answer the questions: *Is this a quality curriculum? On what basis can we say so?*

Faculty rely, in part, upon guidelines and/or criteria for program approval and accreditation when establishing curriculum standards. They might also write standards particular to the school of nursing (e.g., that success rates on NCLEX will exceed national standards [Jacobs & Koehn, 2004]). Consideration should also be given to standards for various curriculum components. For some, such as teaching, the literature is replete with criteria for effective teaching. These can be invaluable in reaching an agreement about school-specific standards. For other components, faculty may have to develop their own standards.

The standards, criteria, and indicators must be specific enough to be understandable and provide direction for data collection and evaluative judgments, while not being too extensive and detailed. Faculty might ask themselves:

- Are the standards, criteria, and indicators consistent with the curriculum intent and with those used by external evaluating agencies?
- Do the number and nature of the standards, criteria, and indicators seem reasonable?

Planning Data Collection

The standards, criteria, and indicators that have been formulated determine which data are necessary for curriculum evaluation. Although a wealth of data might be relevant, only the most pertinent should be assembled. The same data might also provide evidence of the effectiveness of several aspects of the curriculum. For example, student journals can indicate the extent to which course goals are being achieved, as well as provide evidence that evaluation methods are appropriate for the course and curriculum. In planning data collection, faculty need to consider what is reasonable and feasible.

Data Collection Methods

The data collection methods are linked to the evaluation purposes, model selected, and pre-determined standards. Typically, both qualitative and quantitative data are obtained. The methods and tools should allow for a comprehensive evaluation, be understandable and easy to use, cost and time efficient, valid and reliable (if quantitative), and credible (if qualitative).

Quantitative and qualitative data-collection methods and procedures with which most faculty are already familiar can be employed for curriculum evaluation. *Surveys* can be used to assess teachers' and students' level of confidence or satisfaction with the curriculum, their views about specific teaching strategies, infusion of the philosophical approaches into the curriculum, and so forth. *Interviews* (individual or focus group) can reveal quantitative or qualitative data from students, faculty or graduates for similar purposes. Interviews and surveys are also effective in obtaining data from clinicians.

Unstructured observations, and annotations about them, can be useful early in the evaluation process. From these, *structured observation* based on criteria can be planned. For example, observations of students in the clinical area can lead to criteria for structured observations and the acquisition of more specific data about students' clinical abilities and developing attitudes and values. *Anecdotal* notes can be used to record observations related to the goals being evaluated and, when accumulated, can form periodic summative evaluations of student performance (Bourke & Ihrke, 2005; Fitzpatrick et al., 2004). Similarly, peer or expert observation can provide insights into classroom and clinical teaching.

Rating scales, checklists, and self-reports are other means of obtaining data for curriculum evaluation. Rating scales could be used to measure abstract concepts, while checklists can identify expected behaviors or competencies and related student performance. Attitude scales can measure how students and faculty feel about a particular subject or situation, for example, a course or teaching-learning activity. Faculty could use self-reports or journals to record their ideas and insights as they implement the curriculum. Similarly, student narratives can provide information about their reflections, thoughts, fears, goals, progress, successes, and ideas for curriculum improvement.

Data Sources

Data sources include faculty, students, administrators, nurses, and nursing leaders, as well as curriculum and course documents. Student essays, journals, and other assignments can provide valuable insights about their knowledge, attitudes, and experiences. Records, such as student grades, attrition rates, or success rates on licensure examinations are useful for curriculum evaluation. As well, data from formal evaluation processes already in place, such as institution-wide teaching or course evaluations can be used. The use of multiple sources produces a fair and balanced system, with the combination making up for the shortcomings of each (Appling, Naumann, & Berk, 2001).

Scheduling Data Collection

The timing of data collection is important. It should begin with the first courses so that formative evaluation is undertaken concurrently with curriculum implementation. In this way, early decisions arising from formative evaluation can stabilize the curriculum and prevent problems that might occur in courses yet to be implemented.

Some scheduling seems self-evident. For example, student evaluation of courses typically occurs at the completion of each course. However, formal course evaluation mandated by educational institutions is unlikely to address all the questions to which curriculum evaluators seek answers. Therefore, planning for curriculum evaluation should take the timing of additional data collection into account. For example, when is the best time to schedule collection of student data about courses and teaching approaches so students will participate without fear of penalty for unfavorable comments, or without giving up time they feel would be better spent on assignments or studying for examinations? Similarly, it is evident that data collection about graduates' abilities cannot occur until there are graduates, but timing and frequency must be determined.

A reasonable schedule for collecting pertinent data should be developed. The intent is to ensure that data are collected as frequently as necessary to provide an adequate basis for meaningful evaluation, yet not so often that the task is unduly burdensome.

Data Management and Reporting

It is vital that a decision be made about who will have responsibility for data collection, compilation, interpretation, and formulation of judgments. Additionally, there should be consideration of a system to store data and record evaluation deliberations. When regular reporting to external agencies is necessary, accountability for doing so must be established.

As well, a decision should be made about whether data collected for curriculum evaluation will be used for other purposes. If so, who will have access to the data? For example, if teaching or course evaluations beyond standardized institution-wide questionnaires are undertaken, discussion about how the results will be reported and used is necessary. If faculty journals or portfolios are requested, then who will read them and how will they be assessed in relation to the curriculum? Who will receive the results? Will school-specific teaching evaluations be public, if this is not mandated by institutional policies? Will school-specific teaching evaluations be used solely for curriculum evaluation or will they also be used for promotion and tenure purposes? Agreement about these and similar questions should be reached before curriculum evaluation is implemented.

Faculty Deliberations about Data Collection Plans

Planning data collection requires attention to the methods to be employed, the scope of data required, and logistics of the undertaking. When developing a plan for data collection, faculty might consider:

- What data are required to ascertain if standards are being attained?
- How can data be obtained expeditiously?
- When, how, and from whom will data be collected?
- Who will be responsible for developing, pilot-testing, and approving data-collection tools?
- Who will have responsibility for overseeing data collection and analysis?
- How often will data be reviewed and interpreted, so that conclusions can be drawn? Who will participate in this process?
- How will evaluation results be reported? To whom?
- How will evaluation activities, results, and curriculum alterations be documented so that these records can contribute meaningfully to external summative evaluation?

- Will evaluation data be used for faculty evaluation or faculty development purposes?
- What resources are required to conduct these activities?

Planning Evaluation of Curriculum Components

Curriculum Goals

The goals, broadly stated, identify the abilities of graduates and incorporate the philosophical approaches of the curriculum. The complexity of the abilities should be appropriate for the educational level of the program and be consistent with (or exceed) criteria for approval and/or accreditation. If program graduates are to write licensure exams, the curriculum goals should incorporate the abilities expected of new entrants to the profession.

When planning the evaluation of curriculum goals, faculty want to determine if the curriculum goals are appropriate and reasonable, i.e., *are these the right goals?* More specifically, faculty are interested in the extent to which the curriculum goals:

- reflect the practice and standards of the educational institution, higher education, the nursing profession, state or provincial licensing bodies, and approval or accrediting organizations
- are appropriate to the program level
- are unique to the school of nursing

Curriculum Design

When planning evaluation of the curriculum design, the scope of this component becomes evident. The design encompasses the curriculum goals and the configuration of the program of studies (i.e., courses, their sequence, inter-relationships, and mode of delivery). As well, it includes teacher and student activities, and policies governing the curriculum. When planning evaluation of the curriculum design, faculty are interested in the extent to which:

- the curriculum elements fit together
- the design reflects the philosophical approaches and curriculum goals
- the design accounts for the geographical and cultural context of the community
- the configuration of courses supports student achievement of curriculum goals
- there is consistency, congruence, and organization among the courses
- support courses facilitate achievement of curriculum goals and contribute to a well-rounded liberal education

- the necessary pre-requisites are included so students can be successful
- students and faculty believe that the courses are appropriate and logically sequenced

Learning Outcomes

The purpose of all nursing curricula is to prepare students to practice nursing competently. Therefore, it is essential to determine if current students are progressing toward this outcome and if graduates are successful as they begin practice. Evaluation of student learning outcomes is viewed by some as the most important aspect of curriculum evaluation. The over-riding question is: *are students being adequately prepared for professional practice?* Data about the following should be examined:

- success rates on licensure examinations in comparison to provincial, state, or national results
- the extent to which:
  - students are achieving course and curriculum goals
  - students and faculty can articulate philosophical approaches, curriculum goals, and curriculum concepts
  - students can describe how they use curriculum concepts and philosophical approaches in clinical experiences
  - graduates feel ready to begin practice
  - new graduates are successful in their positions

Courses

Evaluation of courses is, in some measure, a microcosm of the evaluation of curriculum goals, design, and outcomes. All aspects of course design and implementation are considered. Faculty might determine the extent to which:

- course goals are appropriate and linked to curriculum goals
- expectations of students are reasonable
- learning activities are consistent with the philosophical approaches and goals
- course activities contribute to students' progress
- course activities suit the delivery mode
- teaching strategies and technologies are effective in facilitating learning
- content is current, research-based, related to other fields of study, and logically organized

- evaluation methods are appropriate in nature and number
- students have achieved course goals
- each course can be justified within the curriculum
- there are redundancies or deficiencies among courses
- each course has been implemented as originally conceived

Teaching Strategies

When planning evaluation of teaching, faculty can be guided by literature that describes effective teaching and lists desirable teacher competencies, behaviors, or characteristics for classroom and clinical courses (Bevis, 2000a, 2000b; DeYoung, 2003; Gignac-Caille & Oermann, 2001; Johnsen, Assgaard, Wahl, & Salminen, 2002; Murray, 2000; Reilly & Oermann, 1999). These descriptions generally address the dimensions of professional competence, relationships with students, personal characteristics, evaluation practices, and teaching skills. Ideas from the literature can be adopted, adapted, or extended to suit the curriculum.

It is wise to remember the recommendation of the National League for Nursing, that ". . . evaluation practices do not inhibit . . . faculty efforts to be creative in their approaches to teaching" (Anonymous, 2004, p. 49). This implies that evaluation standards, procedures, and judgments should be flexible so that teaching strategies are not fixed and unchanging. In general, faculty seek to answer the following questions.

- What is the nature of student-faculty interactions?
- How do students respond to the teaching strategies?
- In what ways have faculty affected students' growth as individuals and future practitioners?
- To what extent:
  - are teaching strategies congruent with the philosophical approaches?
  - do teaching strategies assist students in their progress toward course and curriculum goals?
  - do teaching approaches respect student diversity?
  - are students satisfied with the teaching in the curriculum?
  - do faculty feel satisfied with their teaching?

Student Evaluation Strategies

Appraisal of strategies to evaluate student learning is another important dimension of curriculum evaluation. The evaluation strategies have great significance to students and color their reaction to the curriculum. Questions that might be considered when evaluating these strategies follow.

- What evaluation strategies are used throughout the curriculum? Is there diversity or do a few strategies predominate?
- How do students and faculty perceive the evaluation strategies with respect to diversity, fairness, and flexibility?
- To what extent:
  - are evaluation strategies congruent with the philosophical approaches and goals of the curriculum?
  - do the strategies provide for demonstration of all types of learning?
  - are evaluation strategies varied within a course, semester, and year to accommodate students'
    - diverse ways of knowing
    - academic workloads
    - need for formative and summative feedback
    - desire to have input into their evaluation?
  - do evaluation strategies accommodate faculty members':
    - academic workloads
    - expertise and preferences?

Human and Physical Resources

An important dimension of curriculum evaluation is ascertaining if suitable and sufficient human and physical resources are present. Therefore, when planning curriculum evaluation, faculty formulate questions about the extent to which:

- academic and clinical faculty are sufficient in numbers and academic preparation to offer the curriculum in the manner envisioned
- faculty teaching assignments are aligned with their expertise
- staff numbers, roles, and functions are sufficient to support the curriculum
- offices and meeting rooms are available and adequate
- classrooms are adequate in size, structure, comfort, and appearance
- classrooms and labs are equipped with appropriate and functional technologies
- clinical placements and experiences are sufficient in quality and quantity
- library holdings are sufficient in number, scope, and quality
- material resources are adequate

Learning Climate

The learning climate is the social, emotional, and intellectual atmosphere that exists within the school. It influences the quality of life of students, faculty, and staff. The learning climate is important regardless of the medium through which the curriculum is offered. In planning the evaluation of this aspect of the curriculum, faculty might wish to determine the extent to which faculty and students are satisfied with the:

- learning opportunities available
- setting(s) in which learning occurs
- flexibility in the curriculum
- relationships with one another
- perceived freedom to take intellectual risks and make mistakes without repercussions
- support available when undertaking new challenges
- variety of perspectives in course content, discussion, and readings
- diversity of backgrounds of authors of required texts and readings (Saunders & Kardia, n.d.)
- fostering of responsibility and accountability
- sense of belonging and feeling of community

Policies

Curriculum policies are intended to support students' achievement of curriculum goals while ensuring that academic standards are maintained. Therefore, in reviewing and evaluating curriculum policies, faculty consider whether the policies are appropriate, reasonable, understood by faculty and students, and applied consistently. Evaluators might also wish to ascertain if there have been situations that might indicate a need for new policies.

Faculty Development

Faculty development can initially focus on the purposes and processes of curriculum evaluation. Following this, information about evaluation approaches, standards, criteria, and indicators can be presented. Through discussion, faculty can formulate evaluation questions to be answered about each curriculum component, and determine data collection approaches. Published accreditation or approval guidelines can serve as exemplars during these activities. Having completed all previous aspects of curriculum development, novices will understand the curriculum components, but may need assistance with defining standards and criteria and limiting the extent of data collection. Examples of curriculum data might be provided so faculty can practice interpreting and judging.

Chapter Summary

In this chapter, the definition, purposes, and models of curriculum evaluation are presented. These are followed by ideas about planning the overall curriculum evaluation: establishing standards, criteria, and indicators; and planning data collection. Then, evaluation of individual curriculum components is addressed, with emphasis on evaluation questions that might be considered for each. The curriculum components include goals, design, and outcomes; courses; teaching and evaluation strategies; human and physical resources; learning climate; and policies. Ideas for faculty development are proposed.

Synthesis Activities

As in previous chapters, two cases are presented for review and discussion. The first is critiqued; the second is for analysis. Following the cases are questions for consideration when curriculum evaluation is planned in individual settings.

Parkview Community College Department of Nursing

The nursing faculty of Parkview Community College Department of Nursing have been revising their associate degree nursing curriculum for the purpose of updating, and for the forthcoming accreditation visit. Using their collected reports of periodic formative curriculum evaluations and the annual summative evaluation, faculty have been revising the curriculum over the past 8 months. They are satisfied with their progress. According to all stakeholders, the revised curriculum is complete. Relevant external and internal factors that impinge on the curriculum were taken into account. The reshaped philosophical approaches and goals of the program were aligned with the institution's mission and current health care requirements. As well, the faculty's beliefs and student needs were more clearly articulated.

The Chair, faculty, and other stakeholders have worked together to redesign the overall curriculum and individual courses. This has been a time-consuming undertaking, and all have participated beyond their usual workload to complete the revisions for implementation for the incoming class. They are satisfied that the revised curriculum will enable students to achieve the outcomes, and feel prepared to submit the accreditation self-report in the autumn. The Chair has reminded faculty that evaluation of the revised curriculum should proceed, once it is implemented in the fall term.

Critique Parkview nursing faculty have progressed to the point that they feel they are ready to implement the revised nursing curriculum in the fall, and undergo program accreditation. They are to be congratulated for completing the work in 8 months, and for periodically evaluating the former curriculum. Furthermore, they appear to be a cohesive group, working long hours with the Chair, and agreeing upon the curriculum revisions.

While there is evidence of curriculum evaluation, there is no mention of organized documentation or recording of the evaluation results, nor of how the formative and summative evaluations have shaped the revised curriculum. It also does not appear that thought has been given to establishing a curriculum evaluation subcommittee, or to using a curriculum evaluation model appropriate for the curriculum. An evaluation plan for monitoring the revised curriculum is not evident. This would make one wonder what curricular components will be evaluated, who will do this, how and when it will be done, what tools will be used to collect the data, and if the faculty realize the contributions these data can make to students, faculty, and the curriculum itself. Additionally, a curriculum evaluation subcommittee and/or the faculty should first develop evaluative criteria and indicators, based on an agreed-upon curriculum evaluation model. This approach would be useful in meeting approval and accreditation requirements.

Aurora Borealis University Department of Nursing

Aurora Borealis University is located in the circumpolar region at the border of the Yukon Territory in Canada and Alaska in the United States. It is an unusual institution, jointly administered by Canadian and American educators, with students from the northern regions of both countries. Many courses, even entire programs, are offered through distance education and therefore, few faculty are required to be on-campus. Face-to face programs and courses are offered at the home site, or in communities in Alaska, the Yukon, and Northwest Territories. Courses requiring travel by faculty are typically not offered during the harshest months of November to March.

An upper-division nursing program was developed to meet the needs of the northern regions for nurses. There is a strong emphasis on community-based nursing care, community development, traditional health practices and beliefs of indigenous peoples. The Aurora Borealis nursing program hopes to retain its graduates in the north, since students studying in the "south" generally do not return to their home communities.

Three masters-prepared and one PhD-prepared faculty designed the curriculum to be responsive to the northern context, and to achieve the accreditation standards of the National League for Nursing Accreditation Commission and the Canadian Association of Schools of Nursing. Variations in the program take national differences into account. For example, there are two courses about health care systems, legislation, and policy: one addresses the American context, and the other, the Canadian. Students enroll in the course that matches their national origin.

All non-nursing courses can be completed by distance education from Aurora Borealis or through American and Canadian "southern" universities contracted to provide courses. These courses are all pre-requisite to the upper division nursing courses. In the junior year, nursing theory classes are offered on campus, with concurrent community-based experiences. Hospital-based clinical experience occurs in blocks in May and June, and August and September following the junior year, and again in March of the senior year. A one-month practicum in the site of each student's choice is scheduled for April of the final year. Students graduate in June.

The nursing courses are about to be offered for the first time. In addition to classroom courses, university faculty will provide some direct clinical teaching. Because some clinical experiences are in geographically-dispersed locations, local nurses will assume responsibility for clinical teaching. Clinical teaching workshops have been planned, but only a few nurses are likely to attend. Information about clinical teaching is also provided through printed materials, on the school web site, and by audio tele-conferencing.

Twenty-five students will be admitted to the nursing courses every second year. Therefore, all nursing courses will not have to be offered simultaneously.

Faculty recognize that an evaluation plan should be in place, and evaluation initiated concurrently with curriculum implementation. This seems like a daunting task as they busily prepare the first courses. Nonetheless, they have decided that they will use Stufflebeam's CIPP model, since they believe it will make evident the unusual context of the program.

Questions for Consideration and Analysis of the Aurora Borealis Case

1. Does Stufflebeam's CIPP model seem like a reasonable choice? Why? Which other models would be appropriate?

2. Which data will address each component of the model?

3. Develop a feasible data collection and management plan for this faculty.

4. How should evaluation results be reported?

5. Discuss how planning and conducting curriculum evaluation is hampered or helped by the small number of faculty.

6. What features of the curriculum will likely be of particular interest to external reviewers? How can faculty take these into account in their evaluation plan?

Evaluation Planning Activities for Consideration in Your Setting

Use the following questions to guide your thinking about your plans for curriculum evaluation, whether your curriculum is face-to-face or offered by distance education.

1. For what purposes should curriculum evaluation be planned?
2. Which evaluation model or approaches should be used, and why?
3. Which aspects of the curriculum will be evaluated?
4. What data should be collected, and from whom?
5. How frequently should data be collected?
6. How will data be recorded?
7. What is our plan for interpreting the data and drawing conclusions?
8. How will a record of our evaluation efforts and subsequent curriculum alterations be maintained?
9. What are faculty learning needs in relation to curriculum evaluation?

References

Anonymous. (2004). NLN Statement: Innovation in Nursing Education: A Call to Reform. *Nursing Education Perspectives, 25*(1), 47–49.

Appling, S.E., Naumann, P.L. & Berk, R.A. (2001). Using a faculty evaluation triad to achieve evidence-based teaching. *Nursing and Health Care Perspectives, 22*(5), 247–251.

Applegate, M.H. (1998). Curriculum evaluation. In D.M. Billings & J.A. Halstead (Eds.), *Teaching in nursing. A guide for faculty.* (pp. 179–208). Philadelphia: W.B. Saunders.

Bevis, E. O. (2000a). Teaching and learning: The key to education and professionalism. In E.O. Bevis & J. Watson (Eds.), *Toward a caring curriculum: A new pedagogy for nursing.* (pp. 153–188). Boston: Jones and Bartlett Publishers.

Bevis, E.O. (2000b). Appendix I: Criteria for student-teacher-student interactions. In E.O. Bevis & J. Watson (Eds.), *Toward a caring curriculum: A new pedagogy for nursing.* (pp 379–381). Boston: Jones and Bartlett Publishers.

Bourke, M.P., & Ihrke, B.A. (2005). The evaluation process: An overview. In D.M. Billings & J.A. Halstead (Eds.), *Teaching in nursing. A guide for faculty* (2nd ed.). (pp. 443–464). St. Louis: Elsevier Saunders.

Chavesse, J. (1994). Curriculum evaluation in nursing education: A review of the literature. *Journal of Advanced Nursing, 14,* 1024–1031.

DeYoung, S. (2003). *Teaching strategies for nurse educators.* Prentice-Hall: Upper Saddle River, NJ.

Ediger, J., Snyder, M., & Corcoran, S. (1983). Selecting a model for use in curriculum evaluation. *Journal of Nursing Education, 22,* 195–199.

Fitzpatrick, J.L., Sanders, J.R., Worthen, B.R. (2004). *Program evaluation: Alternative approaches and practical guidelines* (4th ed.). Boston: Pearson.

Gagné, R.M., Briggs, L.J, & Wager, W.W. (1992). *Principles of instructional design* (4th ed.). New York: Harcourt Brace Yovanovich College Publishers.

Gignac-Caille, A.M. & Oermann, M.H. (2001). Student and faculty perceptions of effective clinical instructors in ADN programs. *Journal of Nursing Education, 40*, 347–353.

Guba, E., & Lincoln, Y. (1989). *Fourth generation evaluation.* Newbury Park, CA: Sage.

Herbener, D.J., & Watson, J.E. (1992). Evaluating nursing education programs. *Nursing Outlook, 40*(1), 27–32.

Jacobs, P.M., & Koehn, M.L. (2004). Curriculum evaluation: Who, when, why, how? *Nursing Education Perspectives, 25*(1), 30–35.

Joel, L.A. (2003). *Kelly's dimensions of professional nursing* (9th ed.). New York: McGraw-Hall Medical Publishing Division.

Johnsen, K.O., Assgaard, H.S., Wahl, H.K., & Salminen, L. (2002). Nurse educator competence: A study of Norwegian nurse educators' opinions of the importance and application of different nurse educator competence domains. *Journal of Nursing Education, 4*, 295–301.

Murray, J.P. (2000). Making the connection: Teacher-student interactions and learning experiences. In E.O. Bevis & J. Watson (Eds.), *Toward a caring curriculum: A new pedagogy for nursing.* (pp. 189–215). Boston: Jones and Bartlett Publishers.

National League for Nursing Accreditation Commission, Inc. (2003). *Accreditation manual for post secondary and higher degree programs in nursing.* New York: Author.

Pateman, B., & Jinks, A. (1999). 'Stories' or 'snapshots'? A study directed at comparing qualitative and quantitative approaches to curriculum evaluation. *Nurse Education Today, 19*, 62–70.

Reilly, D.E., & Oermann, M.H. (1999). *Clinical teaching in nursing education* (2nd ed.). Boston: Jones and Bartlett Publishers.

Saunders, S., & Kardia, D. (n.d.) Creating inclusive college classrooms. Center for Research on Learning and Teaching, University of Michigan. Retrieved April 21, 2004 from *http://www.crlt.umich.edu/gsis/P3_1.html*

Stufflebeam, D.L., Madaus, G.F., & Kellaghan, T. (Eds.) (2000). *Evaluation models: Viewpoints on educational and human services evaluation* (2nd ed.). Boston: Kluwer Academic Publishers.

CHAPTER 11

Planning for Successful Curriculum Implementation

Chapter Overview

Planning for successful implementation of a new curriculum requires thought and effort throughout the curriculum development process. Making implementation plans public includes informing stakeholders as the curriculum is developed and introduced. In this chapter, marketing and publicity are described, as are contractual agreements with health care and community agencies and other educational institutions. The logistics of curriculum implementation are discussed, including personnel, scheduling, and phasing out the existing curriculum. Following a discussion of faculty development, synthesis activities conclude the chapter.

Chapter Goals

- Appreciate the planning necessary to implement a new or revised curriculum
- Consider means to inform others, publicize, and market the curriculum
- Review contractual and logistical arrangements essential in curriculum implementation
- Recognize the value of ongoing faculty development for successful curriculum implementation

Making Curriculum Plans Public

Implementation of the new curriculum should not be a surprise to the community. Rather, all who have been involved in and will be affected by the curriculum should be thoroughly prepared for it. Informing others of evolving plans, and attending to details of implementation, must occur simultaneously with curriculum development.

Informing Stakeholders

Previous chapters have referred to the inclusion of stakeholders in curriculum development. In addition to contributing to the creation of a relevant curriculum, their involvement can result in a sense of curriculum ownership and a desire to ensure its successful implementation. To this end, stakeholders can be regular and effective messengers, keeping others apprised of forthcoming changes and their rationale. The stakeholders can help shape the path for a smooth transition from one curriculum to another.

Students Current students should be informed about curriculum plans, as they are naturally interested in the planned curriculum changes and what the changes will mean for them. This information sharing can be accomplished by faculty and by students who are involved in the curriculum development process. These students can be very helpful in explaining and promoting the developing curriculum to their peers. Faculty must also be diligent in these efforts.

The Educational Institution As curriculum development proceeds, consultation with senior administrators and chairpersons of relevant institution-wide committees is ongoing. Keeping these people informed of the developing curriculum can do much to expedite approval. As well, negotiations about support courses and their scheduling must occur before the curriculum is finalized.

Similarly, arrangements for financial resources, student services, library resources, technological support, and so forth must be made before curriculum approval is requested. Assurance about these matters is gained by engaging the directors of these services in discussion early in the curriculum development process. In this way, they can alert the director of the school of nursing, or the curriculum leader, about any anticipated problems, as well attend to financial and personnel implications within their units.

Health Care and Community Agencies Involvement and support of stakeholders outside the educational institution is foundational to a curriculum with a practice component. Steering Committee members serve as ambassadors for the new curriculum to clinical and community agencies. Support from these and other nursing leaders, while essential, may not be sufficient to ensure successful implementation in clinical sites.

Personnel with whom students will be working must be informed of the new curriculum. This can be accomplished, in part, through formal presentations and the provision of written materials. More detailed, small group meetings are also necessary to orient nursing and other staff to the new learning goals and activities that students will pursue. Faculty whose work intersects with clinical personnel have a critical role in this latter activity. Answering questions and allaying any apprehensions that might surface about the curriculum will be helpful in reducing misconceptions.

If placements are planned in agencies where students have not previously had clinical experiences, curriculum orientation will be particularly important. Discussion should focus on students' learning goals and activities; the nature of student interactions with clients and staff; and logistical details. Interpreting the role of nursing and explaining how nursing students will contribute to agency goals and client well being is essential.

Scheduling follow-up meetings at clinical sites to discuss student experiences in the new program can promote successful implementation of the curriculum. These meetings can address:

- what is working well
- concerns expressed by staff and/or students
- appropriate actions to resolve concerns

As well as facilitating learning experiences for students, these meetings can serve several larger purposes. They can:

- demonstrate the educational institution's interest in the views of practicing nurses
- provide an avenue to express appreciation for staff members' involvement in student learning
- bring to light learning experiences not previously considered
- build commitment to student learning

Ongoing Communication   As curriculum development proceeds, regular town-hall meetings with students, nurses, and others interested in knowing about the curriculum will serve to maintain open dialogue and facilitate a feeling of inclusion. Similarly, an electronic newsletter or a regularly updated web site outlining progress and responses to frequently-asked questions will also help make the process transparent and keep interested parties informed about changes.

Marketing

Marketing of the new curriculum to prospective students is fundamental for successful implementation. Many avenues can be used to make the program known and appealing. For example, professionally-designed pamphlets and brochures can be sent to secondary school counselors, and to academic counseling services within the educational institution. As well, face-to-face meetings can be planned with secondary school counselors to inform them about curricular changes and provide opportunities to clarify and update understandings of the profession and changes within.

An attractive, current, and simple-to-navigate web site about the school of nursing, the curriculum, and faculty will market the nursing curriculum to prospective students. Nursing students and faculty can provide valuable advice about important information to include. Within the site, there should be an easy means to contact the school. A prompt, accurate, and friendly response maintains potential applicants' interest in the school. The reply can be electronic or by telephone. A toll-free line would encourage potential applicants to call with questions.

Other effective marketing tools that would appeal to the millennial generation are videos, DVDs, or CD-ROMs that capture attention by portraying the profession, its diverse career opportunities, the school of nursing, and the curriculum, in a dynamic, positive light. Although there are associated costs, these initiatives could stimulate trans-professional linkages by drawing on the expertise of faculty from journalism, business, dramatic and visual arts, and information technology.

University and college academic fairs, nursing education fairs, open-houses, and visits to secondary schools by faculty, students, and recent graduates, are further means to interest prospective students. Community outreach clinics by students and faculty, and spotlights on the school through the press, radio, or television could keep communities informed of the new curriculum. As well, posters on buses, subways, and billboards would place the school of nursing in the public eye.

Co-op opportunities that include attending some nursing classes or laboratory sessions may stimulate interest in the profession for individuals making career decisions. Job shadowing can inform prospective students about the profession and the nursing curriculum. Additionally, short summer programs designed for secondary school students to "be a nurse for a week" could plant the seeds for developing future nurses.

Contractual Agreements

Health Care and Community Agencies

Nursing programs are usually required to have formal agreements with agencies in which students have clinical experience. The educational institution, on behalf of faculty and students, negotiates these affiliation or contractual agreements. Signed copies of the agreements are retained in the nursing school and the agencies providing learning experiences.

Developing working relationships with agency personnel begins with an initial contact with agency staff. Early meetings clarify the nature and goals of the practice experience, as well as faculty and student roles and responsibilities. Agency personnel can explain the requirements of the setting and their expectations for students and faculty. These first meetings provide the basis for establishing a contract or formal agreement, later negotiated by administrative personnel of both settings. The nature of the experience will influence whether a letter of agreement or formal contract is necessary, or indeed, if a letter of agreement in general terms might be followed by a contract with detailed arrangements specified.

Meetings of faculty and agency staff are also necessary to complete the arrangements and address details of the learning experiences. Staff and faculty need to discuss and agree upon:

- numbers and level of students
- goals and nature of the experience
- students' schedule
- faculty members' roles
- staff expectations
- other details important in the experience.

These discussions confirm the appropriateness of prior decisions about the choice of agencies and units by faculty, choices which are linked to learning goals, clients, staff, and resources for students (Goldenberg & Iwasiw, 1988; Reilly & Oermann, 1999).

Legal Areas of Concern Nurse educators are concerned about issues related to student-educational institution relationships, tort liability, and due process (Lessner, as cited in Reilly & Oermann, 1999). The calendar (bulletin) and other school documents, such as the student handbook, represent an agreement between students and the educational institution. In the practice setting, these documents have legal implications as they guide the behavior of students and faculty. Both faculty and students should be familiar with the goals for the clinical experience, guidelines for clinical evaluation and grading, and policies relevant to clinical practice.

The responsibility and accountability of the educational institution, clinical or community agency, faculty, students, and agency staff should be clarified. All matters related to the legal aspects of clinical education should be addressed when contracts are negotiated and arrangements made for student practice.

Insurance Contracts with community and health care agencies generally stipulate that the educational institution must have insurance for student practice. The insurance policies address matters such as harm to clients, faculty and student liability, student injuries, and equipment loss or breakage. These should be made known to faculty and students. Additionally, the educational institution might require that students have malpractice insurance; faculty generally have professional liability insurance.

Additional Considerations Other matters may be addressed in discussions, formal contracts, or letters of agreement between the school of nursing and the health care or community agency. These might include:

- whether the full names of all students and instructors must be specified prior to the experience (O'Connor, 2001)
- the maximum number of students who can be supervised by one instructor (O'Connor, 2001)
- an orientation of faculty and students to agency policies and procedures
- health requirements; CPR and first-aid certification of faculty and students
- whether student experiences will proceed if faculty are absent
- patients' or clients' rights with respect to care by students
- responsibilities of staff in relation to student learning

Other Educational Institutions

Arrangements made with other educational institutions would depend on the nature of the experience. Purchased courses on a fee-for-service basis offered at other institutions may not require a formal contract. Rather, a letter of agreement specifying the arrangements might suffice. However, for partnerships (such as collaborative or consortium) contractual agreements are usually necessary. Responsibilities of all partners for developing, approving, and implementing the curriculum, and for financing, are specified (see Chapter 8).

Logistics

Planning for successful implementation of the nursing curriculum necessitates attention to certain logistics. Success requires a commitment by all stakeholders to the mission of the institution, to the purpose of education in general and nursing education in particular, and to the philosophy and goals of the curriculum. Additionally, there must be sufficient finances and human resources to mount and implement the curriculum. Attention must be given to course scheduling and phasing out the existing curriculum.

Personnel

Faculty Sufficient numbers of qualified faculty to teach the courses is of paramount importance. Nursing deans or directors will need to plan whom to retain, recruit, and appoint. Characteristics to look for in suitable faculty should include knowledge of relevant content, teaching skills, clinical competence (for those assuming clinical teaching responsibilities), effective interpersonal relationships, and personal attributes of effective teachers. Faculty should be assigned to courses on the basis of their expertise and preferences, and contingent upon faculty workload agreements.

Some faculty will probably be required to teach in the existing and new curricula simultaneously, and may feel over-stretched as they strive for excellence in both. The school leader must be cognizant of suitable teaching assignments for individuals and ensure that not too much is expected. Conversely, some faculty may be faced with the prospect of a lightened teaching assignment, or even with no obvious assignment for a semester or an academic year as the new curriculum is being introduced. The school director has the responsibility of ensuring that teaching loads are consistent with workload agreements, that there is a sense of fairness, and that faculty and students are well served in the process.

In the event that additional faculty will be required to "cover" all the courses, they should be hired. As well, adjunct faculty could be engaged for some of the teaching. Inevitably, this would necessitate planning and organizing faculty orientation and development sessions which, in turn, will require the institution to hire consultants or ask experienced and willing faculty to conduct these activities. Attention to faculty turnover, retention, retirement, and renewal is also necessary when implementation of a new or revised curriculum is being planned.

Support Staff Administrative, secretarial, and clerical services must be in place to implement the curriculum successfully. Personnel such as an administrative assistant and/or secretary to the dean or director, secretaries for undergraduate and graduate programs, and staff to manage student clinical placements should be aligned with the needs of the new curriculum.

Scheduling

Most educational institutions require scheduling requests for classrooms, laboratories, and clinical experiences far in advance of the term when they are needed. In view of increasing enrollments in post-secondary institutions and commensurate with decreasing budgets to fund new classrooms and buildings, equitable and careful planning and allocation of space and equipment are necessary. The school of nursing, therefore, must have such data prepared months in advance of the start of the academic year so courses can be timetabled. This may entail prolonged negotiation before classroom and laboratory schedules are finalized.

Scheduling for student clinical experiences can require joint planning with personnel from other programs and institutions. Students in other nursing programs, medicine, physical therapy, occupational therapy, psychology and social work also need practice experiences. Therefore, clinical placement schedules for all these groups must be coordinated for each health care or community agency where learning experiences in the new curriculum will occur.

Phasing Out the Existing Curriculum and Introducing the Changed Curriculum

The process of phasing out the existing curriculum and introducing the changed one requires attention. It is common for experiences in a changed curriculum to be sequenced differently than in the previous one. Accordingly, students in both curricula may require similar classroom courses, and access to the same practice sites, at the same time. This curriculum overlap must be accounted for so that neither group of students feels disadvantaged, and so that clinical sites do not feel overwhelmed by large numbers of students.

In addition to considering faculty workload during curriculum change, thoughtful attention must be given to the sensitivities of students in both the existing and changed curriculum. References by faculty to the *old* and *new* curriculum can heighten feelings. Students enrolled in the current curriculum might feel that their program is outmoded and that faculty interest lies with the revised curriculum. Special attention should be given this group so they do not harbor resentment. In contrast, the first students in the changed curriculum often feel that they are "guinea pigs," an experimental group on which new educational approaches are being tested. This perception may be reinforced by the fact that curricular refinements will occur as a result of their feedback. Faculty should consistently demonstrate confidence in both curricula and convey their belief that all students are receiving an education that will result in competent nursing practice.

Further, faculty must think about how much overlap from the changed curriculum into the existing curriculum is permissible. Understandably, as faculty become immersed in altered philosophical and teaching approaches, they begin to introduce these into the current curriculum. As well, they are influenced by changed curriculum goals and can unintentionally modify their expectations of students in the curriculum that is being phased out. It is worthwhile for faculty to discuss this overlap and come to agreement about the alterations (if any) that will occur so that a suitable balance is achieved between introducing students to new perspectives and maintaining the integrity of the existing curriculum.

Ongoing Faculty Development

Faculty support of the changed curriculum is foundational to success. This support develops as the curriculum is being shaped. As Scales (1985) commented, "Faculty [who have] developed the curriculum . . . will own, honor, and respect the curriculum and will aggressively and actively implement it." (p. 108). The foregoing notwithstanding, active support of faculty is necessary as the changed curriculum is introduced and new teaching approaches adopted. In particular, faculty development activities can support new teaching and evaluation processes that are consonant with the philosophical approaches and goals of the changed curriculum.

Chapter Summary

Successful implementation of a new or revised curriculum requires attention throughout the curriculum development process. Curriculum plans should be public, and this requires intentional efforts to keep all stakeholders informed. Marketing is important, as are contractual agreements with health care, community, and other educational institutions. The logistics of curriculum implementation involve planning for personnel and scheduling, and for phasing out the existing curriculum while introducing a new one. Planning for ongoing faculty development is essential to support the changed curriculum.

Synthesis Activities

In this final chapter, two cases are again presented, one with a critique and the second followed by questions to guide analysis. Then, questions are presented to stimulate thinking when planning curriculum implementation.

Hercal Community College

The faculty of the Hercal Community College Associate Degree Nursing Program have been successful in enrolling increased numbers of first year students. Recruitment and retention of students have been ongoing activities for the past two years, in response to state and national nursing shortages. A revised curriculum, just completed, is to be implemented in September for ninety-five incoming students.

Active advertising for four additional faculty to accommodate the increased enrollment has proven unsuccessful. There are no additional faculty to augment the existing pool of fifteen full-time faculty members. With classes to resume in two months, the Director of the School has called a meeting of faculty to discuss workloads for the forthcoming academic year. Responsibilities for classroom and clinical teaching are to be allocated, with the goal of distributing workloads evenly while remaining within the union contract.

Local clinical agencies have been contacted for clinical experiences. These include one primary care, 300-bed hospital and one 150-bed chronic and rehabilitation institution, where first and second-year students have had clinical experiences caring for senior, middle, and young adults, as well as children. Directors of these agencies are satisfied with previous arrangements, and further discussion was not deemed necessary.

However, in order to accommodate the increased number of students in the clinical areas, the Director and faculty agreed that an experience with healthy school-aged children could be included for first year students, in addition to their clinical experience caring for adult clients. Because of the limited time to plan for this experience, the Director of the

School telephoned the community health nurse manager responsible for school health. The manager agreed to the Director's request for student placement.

Plans for implementation of the revised curriculum are in place. Faculty are determined to demonstrate respect for all students and both curricula. They agreed not to refer to the two curricula as *old* and *new*. Faculty expressed commitment to assist all students to meet curriculum goals and attain professional standards. With the revised curriculum planned, and the existing curriculum ongoing, the faculty are ready to implement the revised curriculum.

Critique The Director and faculty of Hercal Community College Associate Degree Program have done well to complete their revised curriculum. They have increased enrollment in response to the need for more nurses. The faculty have also met to adjust their workloads to "cover" classroom and clinical teaching within the boundaries of their contract. It is apparent that they are a unified, caring group, as exemplified by their commitment to implement the revised curriculum, complete the existing curriculum, treat all students equally, and help them reach curriculum goals. Also noteworthy is the successful working relationship the Director has with the public health nurse manager.

The agreement by the faculty to share the workload, while honorable on the surface, may not, however, be feasible. Increased teaching responsibilities in both curricula could prove onerous over time, and lead to dissatisfaction, if not to ineffective teaching. The Director should hire part-time instructors and clinical teachers, at least for the forthcoming year, and use the two summer months for faculty development activities for these teachers, who may be inexperienced. This investment could motivate these faculty to consider a full-time appointment. Active faculty recruitment efforts should be also undertaken to accommodate future students.

Selecting a new experience for first year students may be appropriate because of increased numbers. However, there has been no meeting with the community health manager and staff to discuss the purpose of the experience (where students have not been before), scheduling, numbers of students, roles and responsibilities of staff, faculty and students. Scheduled meetings to discuss these matters, as well as contractual arrangements between the college and community health agency, should be planned.

Jasmine University School of Nursing

Faculty of Jasmine University School of Nursing have worked diligently to develop a new curriculum. Although they considered the advantages of an upper-division nursing program, they decided to continue with their 4-year integrated curriculum. The new curriculum is based in phenomenology, feminism, and humanism, with a strong emphasis on community-based nursing. However, hospital-based practice remains a feature of the curriculum. Concurrent with the introduction of the new curriculum will be a fifty percent increase in the class size from 100 to 150.

For more than 35 years, university students have had on-campus classes from Monday to Wednesday, with hospital-and community-based clinical practice on Thursday and Friday, during the day. Other nursing programs in the city have had clinical experiences at times other than Thursday and Friday daytime.

As they discuss phasing out the existing curriculum and introducing the new one, faculty identify a significant problem with clinical placements. Currently, fourth-year students have an experience on maternal-infant units in the fall semester. In the changed curriculum, this experience is scheduled in the fall and winter semesters of the second year (75 students in each semester). Both groups have 2 days of clinical experience each week. This means that for 2 consecutive years, 100 fourth-year students and 75 second-year students will need to be placed on the same units on Thursdays and Fridays in the fall semester. In addition, the popularity of home births, discharges from hospital 8–24 hours after delivery, and city-wide hospital restructuring will lead to a 40% decrease in the number of family birthing rooms.

Questions for Consideration of the Jasmine University Case

1. What are the logistical considerations in this case?
2. What options are possible to address this situation?
3. What are the possible implications for students, faculty, and the clinical agency for each of the options proposed?
4. Should faculty reconsider the design of the new curriculum? Justify whether or not they should.
5. In what ways can faculty prevent situations such as this when a new curriculum is being planned and implemented?

Curriculum Implementation Questions for Consideration in Your Setting

The questions below are intended to guide thinking as you plan curriculum implementation.

1. What planning steps are critical for successful curriculum implementation?
2. How can stakeholders be informed of the developing curriculum and implementation plans?
3. How can a smooth transition to the changed curriculum in clinical sites be ensured? How can clinical faculty inform clinicians of the proposed curriculum changes? How else can clinical stakeholders be informed?

4. Who will be responsible for initiating contact and exploring learning opportunities in new practice sites? For initiating contract discussions? For orienting staff to the curriculum and student learning goals?

5. Which marketing strategies could be used? Who will be responsible for them? Who could help with marketing?

6. How can necessary human, physical, and financial resources be ensured to implement the curriculum?

7. Who will be responsible for apprising administrative personnel of the scheduling needs within the new curriculum?

8. What strategies might alleviate student concerns about being learners in a new curriculum? Similarly, how might concerns of students in an existing curriculum be alleviated?

9. What are the plans for phasing out the existing curriculum?

10. Which ongoing faculty development activities should be planned?

References

Goldenberg, D., & Iwasiw, C. (1988). Criteria used for patient selection for nursing students' hospital clinical experience. *Journal of Nursing Education, 27,* 258–265.

O'Connor, A.B. (2001). *Clinical instruction and evaluation. A teaching resource.* Boston: Jones and Bartlett Publishers and National League for Nursing.

Reilly, D.E., & Oermann, M.H. (1999). *Clinical teaching in nursing education.* (2nd ed.). Boston: Jones and Bartlett Publishers.

Scales, F.S. (1985). *Nursing curriculum development, structure, function.* Norwalk: Appleton-Century-Crofts.

Index

progressions policies, 183

progressive theories, 150–151

proposing curriculum possibilities, 115–117

   Poplarfield case study, 126–127

prospective students. *See* students

provincial licensing bodies, goals of, 156

Provus' discrepancy evaluation model, 227

publication, potential for, 46

publicizing curriculum plans, 244–245

publicly voiced criticism, 68

purpose of courses, 194, 210

Q

qualitative data-collection methods, 230

qualitative models of curriculum evaluation, 224

quality standards, influence of, 89, 102. *See also* evaluating curricula

quantitative data-collection methods, 230

quantitative models of curriculum evaluation, 224

quantum leadership style, 30

questioning as teaching strategy, 207

R

race, influence of, 88

range of courses offered, 83

rating scales, 230

re-evaluation of change, 62–63

real-time curriculum delivery, 168

realism, 147

reconstructive theories, 150–151

recordkeeping, 34

reflective journaling as teaching strategy, 207

refreezing phase of change, 60

regulations. *See* policies of education institution

reinforcement management, 64

relational humanism, 150, 153

relationships. *See* collaboration; interpersonal aspects of curriculum development

reluctance to change. *See* resistance to change

remote curriculum delivery, 167–169

   course design, 202–204

   teaching strategies, 204

Renzulli's features evaluation model, 227

reporting, 232

resistance to change, 6, 82. *See also* support for change

   academic freedom, 45, 73

   criticism, identifying, 15–16

   initial, addressing, 12, 15–17

   responding to, 61, 67–73

   workload increase. *See* workload, as barrier

resources

   as contextual factor, 83, 97–98

     Poplarfield case study, 127–133

   course design and, 198

   evaluating, 236

   financial. *See* finances

   human resources (personnel), 83–84, 98

     administrative resources and support staff, 84

     course design and, 198

     evaluating, 236

     informing of curriculum plans, 244–245

     logistics of curriculum implementation, 248–249

     Poplarfield case study, 129–131

   infrastructure of educational institution, 83–86, 98

     Poplarfield case study, 129–133

     teaching strategies, 205–208

   material resources, 198

   physical space, 84, 99

     course design and, 198

     evaluating, 236

     Poplarfield case study, 131

   securing, 45

   teaching strategies, 205–208

   work plan, 36–45

respect, collegiate, 16

responsibilities and roles, 54–55

state boards of nursing, goals of, 156
steering committees, 33
Stenhouse evaluation model, 228
stimulus control, 65
Stonehill University School of Nursing
    (case study), 22
structure of committees, 31–36
structured observations, 230
structures (types) of programs, 167, 197
student conduct guidelines, 183
student presentation as teaching strategy, 207
student services, 86, 100
    Poplarfield case study, 133
students
    assessment of student learning, 197, 208, 212
    curriculum design implications, 184
    engagement of, 204–208
    evaluating, 197, 208, 212
        strategies for, 235–236
    informing of curriculum plans, 244
    learning activities, 197, 201, 212
    participation in curriculum development, 18
    as resource, 84–85, 155
    role in course design, 201
Stufflebeam's CIPP evaluation model, 227
Stufflebeam's educational decision evaluation
    model, 228
subcommittees, 32–33, 40–45
summative curriculum evaluation, 222
support courses, adding to curriculum, 182
support for change, 3, 6, 12. See also resistance
        to change
    academic freedom, 45, 73
    curriculum goals, 155
    faculty role, 61
    how to approach colleagues, 14
support for teaching/learning, 85–86, 99–100,
        121–122, 155
    Poplarfield case study, 132–133
surveys, 95, 230
synchronous curriculum delivery, 168

synthesis of contextual data, 111–123
    administrative issues, 112, 117
        facilitation of curriculum design, 177
        Poplarfield case study, 118–120, 126–141
    determining directions and outcomes,
        121–122
    examination and integration, 113–114
    faculty development for, 123
    human implications of curriculum design,
        184
    limitations, identifying, 112, 116
        Poplarfield case study, 118–120, 126–141
    proposing curriculum possibilities, 115–117

T

task forces, 32–33, 40–45
tasks of participants. See responsibilities and
        roles
teachers. See faculty
teaching approaches, 57–58
teaching assignments, curriculum design and,
        184
teaching strategies, 195–196, 204–208, 212
teaching support, resources for, 85–86, 99–100,
        121–122, 155
    Poplarfield case study, 132–133
technical evaluation of curricula, 226
technology resources, 84, 90
television-based curriculum delivery, 168
terminal objectives, 154. See also goals of
        curriculum change
theoretical nursing frameworks, 173
theories of change, 60–66
theories of learning, 148
theory-based curriculum organization, 173
think-pair-share as teaching strategy, 207
third-generation evaluation models, 226
time (duration) of curriculum, 167
timeframe and scheduling, 18–20
    curriculum implementation logistics, 249
    data collection, 231